Handbook of Medical English Usage

Handbook of Medical English Usage

with definitions and examples

Simo Merne, MA

Foreword by

Dr Clifford Hawkins
Honorary Consultant Physician, Postgraduate Centre, Queen Elizabeth Hospital, Birmingham

Heinemann Professional Publishing

Heinemann Medical Books
An imprint of Heinemann Professional Publishing Ltd
Halley Court, Jordan Hill, Oxford OX2 8EJ

OXFORD   LONDON   MELBOURNE   AUCKLAND

First published 1989

British Library Cataloguing in Publication Data
Merne, Simo
  Handbook of medical English usage.
  1. Medicine. Terminology
  I. Title
  610′.14
  ISBN 0–433–21250–0

Typeset by Wilmaset, Birkenhead, Wirral,
and printed and bound in Great Britain by
Biddles Ltd, Guildford and King's Lynn

To Märtha, Markus and Marina

Contents

Foreword

Learning from one's mistakes is called experience but learning from the experience of others is less painful. Hence anyone wishing to become proficient in medical English should welcome this book, for it is written by an author whose mother tongue is not English, so he has faced all the problems. Three stages are necessary before success is achieved: first, learning English words, grammar and syntax; secondly, knowing the technical words of medicine – which is not so difficult as many, derived from Latin or Greek, are international; thirdly, understanding words that every profession adopts to use in a special way. The last is an area where failure often occurs because the student has no guidance. This novel annotated dictionary fills this gap.

A good style of writing can be defined as the maximum amount of information conveyed in the minimum number of words written in a pleasing way. Most authors have to edit and rewrite their scripts, often several times, even when using their native language. Clear writing is achieved by deleting all unnecessary words and super-fluous phrases. The author draws attention to this with numerous examples, recommending 'because' instead of 'due to the fact that' and 'probably' rather than 'there can be little doubt that'. Simple words are preferable to long, polysyllabic and pompous-sounding ones; instances given in this book are 'leg' rather than 'lower extremity' and 'show' instead of 'exhibit'. I am also pleased that he advises that the simple word 'before' should usually be used instead of the more pretentious 'prior to'. The appendix provides a check list for writers.

Good taste in using words is difficult to define and especially difficult for those who do not know the language. 'Woman' is rightly suggested rather than 'female' and 'patient' in preference to 'case', although there are, of course, exceptions to those, and to all rules. Guidance is also given about the customary way of expressing thanks under 'acknowledge'. The selection of words that have a similar meaning (synonyms) together with some that are opposite in sense (antonyms) helps the writer to avoid too much repetition.

This book is an invaluable vade-mecum for those who are learning medical English and for anyone who intends to write an article or address a meeting.

Clifford Hawkins Honorary Consultant Physician, Postgraduate Centre, Queen Elizabeth Hospital, Birmingham

Preface

The purpose of this handbook is to show, by means of practical examples, how General English (GE) words and phrases are used in written Medical English (ME). Thus, it attempts to bridge the gap between general dictionaries and standard medical dictionaries. It is an alphabetical glossary of over 2400 headwords with definitions and over 4000 examples of usage. The book is intended for those who take a special interest in English medical writing – medical research workers, doctors, medical students and translators.

The book is based on my 15-year experience as a lecturer of English for Medical Purposes at the School of Translation Studies, University of Turku, Finland, and as a freelance translator and language consultant for medical researchers and pharmaceutical manufacturers. Over these years I have come to recognize the complexities of ME, especially from a non-native writer's viewpoint. Even native professionals sometimes have divergent opinions on ME usage. However, there does seem to be a central body of English language features common to medical authors. It is these typical words and phrases with which this handbook deals.

The emphasis is not on definitions but on the usage pattern of important 'non-technical' or 'semi-technical' words that frequently occur in medical reports. 'Technical' words, more appropriately dealt with by medical dictionaries, have been included only if they are associated with a special language feature – semantic or syntactic.

The entries fall into the following groups:

1. Words referring to diseases, their signs and symptoms, e.g. attack, coma, deteriorate, frank, generalized, herald, irreversible, relapse.
2. Words referring to treatment, e.g. alleviate, hospitalize, infuse, operation, referral, sample, theatre.
3. Words referring to study design, e.g. cross-sectional, prospective, protocol, screening.
4. Words from related disciplines, chemistry, physics, statistics, etc., e.g. absorb, bias, prevalence, significance.
5. Common connective words in scientific texts, e.g. apply, compensate, differ, influence, sustain, and their derivatives.
6. Words that are frequently used in the evaluation of results, e.g. agreement, correlation, frustrating, intersubject, progress, rewarding.

7. Words referring to medical communication, e.g. authority, circularize, information, notify, postulate, report.

These groups include GE words that have a special ME meaning, e.g. admission, follow, history, negative, trial, visualize.

The examples originate from medical articles written by British or American authors for leading medical journals. They do not necessarily reflect current medical opinion. Much of the original material has been abbreviated or otherwise modified to save space and to emphasize the relevant features. The users should study the examples and then apply their observations to their own writing. The handbook describes rather than prescribes medical English usage. Therefore, the inclusion of a word in the glossary should not simply be regarded as a recommendation for its use. Some recommendations have been given in the form of notes, e.g. 'simpler':, 'rare' or '*Note:*'. ME style manuals warn about such expressions as 'exhibit' (= show), 'prior to' (= before) or 'perform' (= do, carry out etc.). However, very much depends on the communicative situation. Good medical writing, as seen in the *British Medical Journal* and the *New England Journal of Medicine*, for example, is not based on rigid language prescriptions but on clear and concise expression.

The appendix at the end of the book lists expressions that are usually ambiguous, clumsy, pompous or vogue words and therefore to be avoided.

Although I have made every effort to include the most important features of general ME phraseology, readers will no doubt notice omissions, inadvertent or intentional, and also errors of which they would like to notify the author. Any constructive comments are welcome.

I wish to thank my colleague Jacqueline Välimäki, University of Turku, as well as Joan Maclean, Edinburgh University, and Dr Chris Sinclair for their insightful and helpful comments during the laborious final stages of manuscript preparation. Dr Clifford Hawkins of the Postgraduate Centre at Queen Elizabeth Hospital, Birmingham, explained many medical facts to me and kindly wrote the foreword. The World Health Organization gave me permission to use some of their basic health term definitions. I also acknowledge the financial support of the Academy of Finland and the Turku University Foundation.

Turku, Finland
April, 1988

Abbreviations and Other Conventions

–	example(s)
←→	opposite(s)
/word 1/word 2/	synonyms
(word)	1. an explanation 2. a common word in this context 3. a common word in this ME context 4. a word that can be missed out.
AE	American English
BE	British English
GE	General English
ME	Medical English
abbr.	abbreviation
adj.	adjective
adv.	adverb
adv. comp.	adverb comparative form
n.	noun
prep.	preposition
pron.	pronoun
rel. pron.	relative pronoun
v.	verb
vi.	intransitive verb (= a verb that does not require a direct object)
vt.	transitive verb (= a verb that usually requires a direct object)

He, she and they in the examples refer to patients.
I/we: doctors.
Any names of research workers are fictitious. No literature sources have been given.
British spelling has been preferred to American spelling where only one is given.

A

abandon *vt.* to give up (completely)

We abandoned the procedure because of its high mortality.

abate *vi.* to (cause to) decrease or lessen (often: from an excessive level)

Bed rest is necessary until the severity of the symptoms has abated.

abatement *n.* a decrease or lessening of the severity of signs and symptoms

The abatement of fever.

Compare: alleviation, remission

aberration *n.* a defect, anomaly

Chromosomal aberrations.

The surgical correction of anatomical aberrations.

adj. aberrant

Compare: abnormality, anomaly

ability *n.* the quality or state of being able

The ability of the liver to desaturate fats.

Compare: capacity

abnormal *adj.* different from the normal, unusual, disease-associated

An abnormal skull radiograph.

A painless swelling of the right testis was the only abnormal finding.

abnormality *n.*

1. the quality or state of being abnormal

Abnormalities /in/of/ bowel function.

2. an abnormal finding

He had an abnormality of the upper lobe of his left lung.

Compare: anomaly

abolish *vt.* to remove by treatment

A hypnotist abolishes pain by suggestion.

n. abolition

abort *n.* rarely: termination of pregnancy (= ME abortion)

abort *vt.* to interrupt, stop at an early stage

These attacks can be avoided or aborted by rest.

To abort a pregnancy.

abortion *n.* the termination of a pregnancy before the fetus has attained viability, i.e. become capable of independent extra-uterine life (WHO 1)

Elective abortion, therapeutic abortion: legal ⟷ illegal abortion.

Induced ⟷ spontaneous abortion.

abortive *adj.*

1. not fully developed

An abortive attack of a disease.

Abortive or mild non-paralytic poliomyelitis.

2. unsuccessful, interrupted

An abortive attempt.

abrupt *adj.* very sudden

The abrupt onset of disease.

abruptly *adj.* in an abrupt manner

His disease began abruptly.

absence *n.* the state of being absent, lack of

The /absence/unavailability/ of obstetric data on a patient.

Renal glycosuria is often found in the absence of any other detectable renal damage.

absent *adj.* not present

The deep tendon reflexes were absent at the ankles.

absorb *vt.* to take or suck in or up, to incorporate

The drug is /rapidly/readily/ absorbed from the gut.

To absorb well, completely ⟷ poorly.

Compare: adsorb, take up

absorption *n.* the process of absorbing or being absorbed

The absorption of glucose into the circulation.

abstain *vi.* to give up (temporarily or completely)

He abstained from smoking tobacco = he stopped smoking *or* he refrained from smoking.

Compare: stop

abstention *n.* giving up or refraining from

They reported complete abstention from smoking.

Compare: cessation

abstract *n.* a short summary, often placed at the beginning of a medical researcher's report

abuse *vt.* to put to wrong use

To abuse drugs.

abuse *n.* wrong use

Alcohol abuse; drug abuse = non-medical use of drug(s).

Child abuse = physical, emotional or sexual injury to a child caused by an adult.

Compare: misuse

abuser *n.* one who abuses

He was identified as an alcohol abuser.

accelerate *vi. vt.* to (cause to) occur more quickly

His pulse accelerated.

The treatment accelerates ulcer healing.

Opposites: decelerate, retard, slow

Compare: speed

acceleration *n.* the act or action of accelerating

The acceleration of the pulse.

accentuate *vt.* to intensify, to make more severe

His haemoglobulinaemia was accentuated during sleep.

Compare: emphasize

accept *vt.*

1. to take, receive

To accept patients for treatment.

The pylorus accepted the endoscope without evidence of stenosis.

Opposite: reject

2. to receive as valid, with approval

This hypothesis has been widely accepted.

We accepted that giving two drugs was adequate treatment.

acceptability *n.*

1. satisfactoriness

The acceptability of a theory.

2. tolerability

The acceptability of a treatment to a patient.

acceptable *adj.*

1. satisfactory

An acceptable suggestion.

2. tolerable

The new drug is acceptable to patients and carries only a low risk of side-effects.

Opposite: unacceptable

acceptance *n.* approval, favourable reception

This method has achieved/gained general/wide acceptance

This technique seems to improve patients' acceptance of an ileostomy.

accepted *adj.* commonly approved

No universally accepted treatment exists for Reye's syndrome.

Our observations may be contrary to the accepted belief.

access *n.* the act of entering, entrance

Bacteria had gained access to the circulation through the lung.

They have access to medical care = medical care is available.

This drug prevents the dietary contents from having access to the inflamed gut.

accessibility *n.* ease of approach

The accessibility of an organ for examination.

accessible *adj.* capable of being reached
>The lesion was accessible to the bronchoscope.
>The tissue was accessible for biopsy, surgery.

accident *n.* an unexpected, unplanned occurrence which may involve injury (WHO 1)
>She sustained severe injuries in the accident.
>Note: a cerebrovascular accident = the stroke syndrome
>*adj.* accidental

accommodation *n.* adjustment
>Accommodation to an altered physiological state.
>The accommodation of the pupils to light.
>*v.* accommodate (to)

accompany *vt.* to occur together with
>Hypertension sometimes accompanies hyperparathyroidism.
>This treatment is accompanied by several side-effects.
>*Compare*: attend, associate

accord *vi.* to be in agreement
>Our observations /accord/usually: are in agreement/ with those of other workers.

accord, accordance *n.* agreement
>Our findings are in complete /accord/accordance/ with previous reports.

account for *v.* to explain
>A virus infection accounted for these symptoms.

accumulate *vi. vt.* to increase in amount
>Bile accumulates in the gall bladder.
>*n.* accumulation

accuracy *n.* precision
>The predictive accuracy of a diagnostic technique.
>The test has an accuracy of 98%.

accurate *adj.* precise
>An accurate diagnosis, accurate results.
>*Opposite*: inaccurate

ache *n.* continuous pain
>A right-sided headache developed.
>He had been suffering from headaches for two years.
>The ache fluctuated in its intensity.
>The aches and pains of old age.
>*v.* ache

achieve *vt.* to accomplish, attain
>To achieve analgesia, high blood steroid concentrations, control of fits, recovery, results by treatment, reversal of renal failure.
>*n.* achievement

acknowledge *vt.* to express gratitude for

I acknowledge the generous grant of the Green Foundation.

I gratefully acknowledge the receipt of funds for research from the Green Foundation.

I should like to acknowledge my debt to . . .

I take pleasure in acknowledging my thanks to . . .

Acknowledgement patterns with thank or thanks:

I should particularly like to thank . . .

I wish to thank . . .

I would like to thank them for cooperation, expert technical assistance, financial help, helpful criticism, helpful suggestions, secretarial help, the statistical analysis, typing the manuscript, valuable discussions.

My special thanks go to . . .

Acknowledgement patterns with grateful or gratitude:

I also have to express my gratitude to . . .

I am most grateful to Professor Hill for his confidence in the project, his generous contribution, permission to report on his patients, the use of his laboratory . . .

n. acknowledgement

acquire *vt.* to come to have

AIDS is usually acquired through a sexual contact.

Hospital-acquired infections ⟷ infections acquired in the community.

An acquired ⟷ congenital disease.

Compare: contract

acquisition *n.* the act of acquiring

The acquisition of an infection.

act *vi.*

1. **act on** = to have an effect on

The drug acts rapidly, promptly, on the central nervous system.

Compare: affect, influence

Opposite: counteract

2. **act as** = to serve the function of

The glycogen in the liver /acts/serves/ as a store of carbohydrate.

action *n.*

1. the effect of a substance on another, on a patient

The drug appears to /have/possess/ an unexpected depressive action.

The desired actions of this drug are exerted primarily on the liver = the drug acts primarily on the liver.

The mechanism of action of this drug is not known.

Compare: activity, effect, efficacy
2. the way in which a part of the body works
The action of the heart.

active *adj*. characterized by action
Active leukaemia ⟷ leukaemia in remission.
The active drug ⟷ placebo.
Opposite: inactive

activity *n*.
1. action, effect
The therapeutic activity of a drug in a disease.
2. functions
Metabolic activity = metabolism.
3. pursuit(s) in which a person is active
He was able to return to his full range of normal activity.
The activities of /daily/normal/ life.

acute disease *n*. some authors maintain that an *acute* illness usually consists of a single episode of fairly short duration from which the patient returns to normal activity, whereas a *chronic* illness is one of long duration in which the patient is permanently incapacitated to a more or less marked degree (WHO 1)
An acute infection frequently has a sudden onset and a finite duration.
Acute anaemia; acute asthma = an acute exacerbation of asthma.
Compare: chronic

adapt *vt*. to make suitable for new circumstances
The body adapts itself to these environmental changes.

adaptable *adj*. capable of adapting oneself
An adaptable organism.

adaptation *n*.
1. the act or action of adapting, the state of being adapted
The menopause may be an adaptation response to ageing.
The salt content of sweat falls on adaptation to a hot climate.
Compare: accommodation, adjustment
2. slight change, modification
The adaptation of a technique for a purpose.

adaptive *adj*. marked by adaptation
Adaptive processes.

add *vi. vt*.
1. *vt*. to unite in order to bring about an increase
Bulk is added to the diet by the addition of extra fruits.
Dermatitis is reversed with added linoleic acid (= if the acid is added to the diet).
2. *vi*. to increase

These new areas of occlusion add to circulatory resistance.

addict *n.* a person who is addicted

A drug addict = a person who is dependent on a drug.

Compare: abuser

addicted *adj.* dependent

To become addicted to a drug.

addiction *n.* dependence

The term *drug dependence* should replace the terms *drug addiction* and *drug habituation*, the term *addiction-producing drug* (along with *habit-forming drug*) should now give place to *dependence-producing drug* (WHO 1).

additional *adj.* in addition, added

Prophylactic antibiotics may provide additional protection for the patient undergoing hysterectomy.

additive *adj.* characterized by addition

The effect of the drug may be additive with other depressants.

additive *n.* a substance added to another in small quantities to improve its properties

This food product contains no additives.

address *vt.* to deal with

This study addresses the problem of fatal asthma.

adhere *vi.*

1. to stick to

Polysaccharides adhere to the tooth surface.

2. to follow closely

To adhere to the study protocol.

adherence *n.* the act or quality of adhering

This method requires /strict/stringent/ adherence to rigidly standardized assay conditions.

adhesion *n.*

1. the act or state of adhering

The adhesion of the inflamed bowel to the bladder.

2. the pathological connection of normally separate tissues, usually as a result of inflammation

The inflamed abdominal organs had become bound by adhesions.

adjacent *adj.* located near, adjoining

The tissue adjacent to the dissected specimen.

adjunct *n.* an auxiliary agent in treatment

A helpful adjunct to treatment.

Immunological testing is a useful and rapid adjunct to neuropathological examinations.

Compare: adjuvant

adjust *vt.*

1. to bring factors of a study to a true relative position

The hydrometer results were adjusted for temperature.

2. to adapt

To adjust drug dosages to the patients' requirements.

adjustment *n.* the act, process or result of adjusting

There was an independent association between cigarette smoking and blood lead concentrations after adjustment for other factors.

The adjustment of acid–base balance to normal.

Compare: adaptation

adjuvant *adj.* aiding

Adjuvant measures.

adjuvant *n.* an agent that improves the efficacy of another treatment

Chemotherapy was given as an adjuvant to surgery.

administer *vt.* to give as a treatment

Intravenously administered gamma globulin.

The drug was administered before meals.

Compare: give

administration *n.* the act or process of administering

The peak concentration occurred at three hours after ad-·ministration of the drug.

admission *n.*

1. acceptance of a subject to a study

Opposite: exclusion

2. the acceptance of a person by a hospital as an inpatient (WHO 1)

Admission to hospital (BE) = admission to the hospital, hospitalization (AE).

Bronchoscopy can be carried out without (hospital) admission.

Urgent (hospital) admission was required.

Admission to intensive care.

Admissions to services, e.g. surgical admissions.

admit *vt.*

1. to confess

He admitted (to) taking 30 tablets of brewer's yeast a day.

Opposite: deny

2. to permit to enter (hospital)

He was admitted for drug withdrawal, oxygen treatment.

He was admitted in terminal renal failure.

adopt *vt.* to bring into use

Conservative measures were adopted = plainly: the patient was treated conservatively.

n. adoption

adsorb *vi. vt.* to form a thin layer attached to the surface of a solid or a liquid
To adsorb onto a surface.
Compare: absorb
n. adsorption

adult *adj.n.* fully developed, grown-up
The study was carried out in adult rats.
This effect was also seen in adults.

advance *n.* development
Advances in computed tomography lessen the need for many invasive procedures.
With the advance of plastic surgery, amputation is now much less needed.
Compare: progress

advance *vi. vt.*
1. *vi. vt.* to move forward
To advance a catheter into a vein.
2. *vi.* to proceed
The cancer had advanced uncontrollably.
3. *vt.* to propose
To advance a theory.

advanced *adj.* being far along in development
Surgical treatment was useful in our advanced cases.

advantage *n.* superiority (of position or condition), merit
The therapeutic advantage of one treatment over another.
This method offers no advantage over skin testing.
advantage $\longleftrightarrow$ disadvantage.
adj. advantageous

advent *n.* arrival, introduction (of something important)
The advent of this method has provided an accurate means of visualizing the adrenal gland.
With the advent of sensitive methods, studies of the absorption of this agent are now possible.
Compare: introduction

adventitious *adj.* additional to normal, extra
Adventitious sounds were heard over the lungs.

adverse *adj.* unfavourable, antagonistic
Adverse reactions to a treatment $\longleftrightarrow$ beneficial effects of a treatment.
An adverse reaction to a drug is one that is noxious, is unintended and occurs at doses normally used in man (WHO 1).
Smoking is considered to be adverse to human longevity.
Compare: side-effects

advice *n.* recommendation

The drug was given on the advice of the physician.

To follow, give advice.

advise *vt.*

1. to give advice, recommend

Contraceptives were advised for these patients.

The couple were advised against pregnancy.

To advise the patient /to use a drug/ $\longleftrightarrow$ /against the use of a drug/ about a treatment.

We advised him that he should stop using this drug.

2. to inform

We advised him of the poor prognosis of the disease.

Note: well-advised (=prudent) and ill-advised (=unwise)

advocate *n.* one who advocates

An advocate of a method, theory, treatment.

Compare: proponent

advocate *vt.* to speak in favour of

To advocate a method, theory, treatment.

affect *vt.* to have an effect on

Age and sex affect resistance to tuberculosis.

affinity *n.* attraction

The /strong/high/ $\longleftrightarrow$ /weak/low/ affinity of a substrate for an enzyme.

Compare: predilection

afflicted *adj.* severely affected

Afflicted with rash.

aftercare *n.* management after the active, curative stage of treatment

age *n.* the period of time that a subject has lived; a period of human life

Albumin levels tend to fall in old age.

Patients /under or above the age of 65/under or above 65 years of age

Since age 18 = since the age of 18.

The baby was small for gestational age.

The patients ranged in age from 14 to 65 years.

The symptoms increased with age.

This disease /is seen/occurs/ at any age.

Age-associated disease.

Note: **young age** is not idiomatic.

aged *adj.*

1. of the stated number of years

We studied three men aged 25, 32 and 52.

2. the aged = elderly people

Senile dementia is a common disease in the aged.

ag(e)ing *adj.* becoming older

An ageing population.

ag(e)ing *n.* the process of becoming older

The central concept of ageing is loss of adaptability of an individual organism with time.

agent *n.* a substance with a certain effect

A disease-causing agent/a pathogenic agent/a pathogen.

The offending agent, the chemical that caused his dermatitis.

This drug was the chief agent for the treatment of anxiety.

aggravate *vt.* to make worse

Hypertension aggravates other disorders arising from diseased arteries.

To aggravate pain.

n. aggravation

Compare: deteriorate, worsen

aggressive *adj.*

1. rapidly invasive

The biological behaviour of a thyroid tumour is not aggressive.

2. marked by drastic measures, very intensive

An aggressive surgical policy was adopted in the management of bleeding peptic ulcers.

These symptoms are indications for aggressive treatment.

agree *v.* to be similar to

Our findings agree with previous reports.

Most surveys agree on an incidence close to 20%.

These two studies agree in showing that . . .

Compare: coincide

agreed *adj.* unanimous

Physiologists are not agreed as to the cortical terminus for the pain fibres.

agreement *n.* the state of being similar or consistent

Good agreement was obtained between the two tests.

These results are in agreement with those of previous studies.

Compare: accord, concert, conformity, consensus, keeping, line

aid *vt.* to help, have a beneficial effect on (particularly in AME)

Topical medications /aid/plainly: are useful for/ superficial lesions.

Compare: help

aid *n.* a device, method etc. that is helpful

A diagnostic /aid/tool/, a hearing aid.

Surgery has been used as an aid in the management of pneumothorax.

This kit is a quick aid to diagnosis.
Compare: tool

ailment *n.* a general term for a (mild) pathological condition particularly before diagnosis
Compare: disease, disorder, illness, sickness

aim *vt.* to direct at
The treatment (was) aimed at alleviating the gastric symptoms.

aim *n.* a purpose
The /aim/purpose/ of a study.

airway *n.* an air passage (to or in the lungs)
To create an /airway/air passage.
To ensure airway maintenance.
To establish an emergency airway.
To maintain an adequate airway.
To secure a clear airway with an oral tube.

alert *adj.* watchful
In this patient we were alert for acute renal failure.
Neurological examination showed that the patient was alert and oriented.
This condition should keep the physician on the alert.

alert *vt.* to warn
We hope our report will /alert others to the risk/ make others aware of the risk

alertness *n.* the state of being alert
Ambulatory patients given sedative hypnotics should be warned to avoid activities which require mental alertness, judgement and physical coordination.

all *pron.* every member of a group
All patients (enrolled in the study) underwent this operation.
All 18 controls were symptom-free.

allay *v.* to make less
To allay a patient's anxiety.
Compare: alleviate

allergic *adj.* hypersensitive (to an antigen)
He was allergic to penicillin.
n. allergy (to)

alleviate *vt.* make less
To alleviate complaints, pain, suffering.
n. alleviation
Compare: mitigate, palliate, relieve

allocate *vt.* to give as a share
Patients were allocated randomly /into/to/ two groups, to receive either oxygen or air.

Compare: allot, assign, divide

allot *vt.* to allocate

This brain area is allotted to memory.

To allot subjects to groups.

Compare: allocate, assign

allow *vt.*

1. to permit (an action)

Hospital personnel with active infection should not be allowed to be in contact with patients.

2. to make possible (an action)

The new method has allowed comparison of the two treatments.

Compare: permit

alone *adv.* by itself (placed after the word to which it refers)

Penicillin alone or in combination with other drugs.

Examples of synonymous phrases:

As a single agent /singly/: the drug was used as a single agent or in combination with other hypotensive drugs.

By itself: the drug used by itself has been shown to reverse thiazide-induced hypokalaemia.

On its own: a pure anxiolytic used on its own.

alter *vt.* to make different

The dosage regimen was altered.

Compare: change

alteration *n.* change

Age-related alterations in metabolism.

alternate *adj.* every second one

Alternate day treatment.

adv. alternately

alternate *vi. vt.* to use or occur alternatively with

The antacid may be alternated with milk every hour.

alternative *adj.* providing a choice

We should develop less expensive alternative dopamine agonists.

adj. alternatively

alternative *n.* something that provides a choice

Alternatives are available to this treatment.

ambient *adj.* in the immediate surroundings

Ambient air contains a variety of organic particles.

ambulant *adj.* able to walk

Ambulant/ambulatory/ ⟷ bedridden, (mainly AE) recumbent patients.

Compare: ambulatory

ambulatory *adj.* able to walk

Ambulatory care = care provided to patients who are not confined to bed (WHO 1).

He was observed on an ambulatory basis.

Compare: ambulant

ameliorate *vi. vt.* to improve

This drug ameliorates hyperthyroidism.

Opposite: deteriorate

Compare: alleviate, improve

amelioration *n.* improvement

Amelioration or removal of risk factors can reduce the likelihood of recurrence of phlebitis.

amenable to *adj.* treatable by

The lung segment was amenable to surgical repair.

Compare: remediable, treatable

amount *n.* extent, quantity

In starvation free fatty acids are produced in large amounts.

amplify *vt.* to make (even) greater

Abnormally great environmental challenges may amplify the effects of ageing.

anaesthesia *n.* loss of feeling or sensation

Biopsy may be carried out under local or general anaesthesia.

anaesthetist (BE), **anesthesiologist** (AE) *n.* a doctor specializing in anaesthesia

analogous *adj.* similar

Resistance to anticancer drugs may be transferred by a process that is analogous to the transfer of antibiotic resistance between cells.

analyse (BE), **analyze** (AE) *vt.* to examine in detail

They were analysed for heparin concentrations by this assay.

analysis *n.* detailed examination

Biochemical analyses were made on urine samples.

This view does not stand up to critical analysis.

To subject a specimen to analysis.

Urine analysis = urine test = urinalysis.

anamnesis *n.* a case history of a patient, history

The word is hardly ever used in English. Use **(case) history.**

anecdotal *adj.* of a case report lacking sufficient evidence or data (obtained from controlled studies)

Anecdotal evidence suggests that children with acute viral croup benefit from a warm, humid environment.

Some journals publish anecdotal reports of adverse drug reactions.

anergic *adj.* suffering from decrease or absence of immunity

He was anergic to a variety of skin test antigens.

anergy *n.* the state of being anergic
Anergy to tuberculin.

announce *vt.* to point to, to indicate in advance
Subacute cord compression is announced by local back pain.
Compare: precede

anomaly *n.* abnormality
A metabolic anomaly = a metabolic abnormality.
Behaviour anomalies.
adj. anomalous

antagonist *n.* a substance that opposes the action of another
Adrenalin is a pharmacological antagonist /to/of/ the effects of
chemical mediators on smooth muscles.

antecedent *adj.* coming or occurring before
An antecedent infection.
Compare: previous

antedate *vt.* to be earlier
These lesions antedated his septicaemia.
Compare: precede

antibody *n.* a substance produced to interact with an antigen
Antibodies /to/(directed) against/ a virus.

anxiety *n.* an intense feeling of apprehension, uneasiness and fear
as a conscious reaction to an unconscious stimulus
adj. anxious

apparatus *n.* organs
The respiratory apparatus.

apparent *adj.* evident, obvious
Clinically apparent skin lesions.
Fever without apparent cause.
Treatment with apparent benefit.
Opposite: inapparent

appear *vi.*
1. to come into sight
The characteristic rash of measles appears three to five days
after onset of symptoms.
2. to seem
These cells appear mature.
It appears from these observations that . . . = (shorter:) These
observations suggest that . . .

appearance *n.*
1. the process or act of appearing
The appearance of a virus in the blood.
2. outward aspect
The radiological appearance of an obstruction.
These cells had a mosaic appearance.

applicable *adj.* that can be applied

This treatment is applicable to several types of cancer.

application *n.*

1. use

The application of electroconvulsive treatment.

This method has found increasing application in the diagnosis of several disorders.

2. putting of one thing on to another

The application of an ointment (on) to the skin.

apply *vi. vt.*

1. *vi.* to be relevant, to have a valid relation

The same finding applied to all women in our series.

2. *vt.* to bring into use, to put on

To apply a principle to practice, medicine to a wound.

To apply pressure to the bleeding point.

appraisal *n.* assessment

He was given a realistic, honest, factual appraisal of the severity of the condition.

appreciable *adj.* great enough to be considered

Appreciable differences.

Compare: considerable

appreciably *adv.* quite considerably

The drug appreciably reduces the acidity of gastric contents.

Note: **appreciably** may sometimes be missed out.

approach *n.* avenue, method, procedure

This technique /provides/is/ a new approach to the management of asthma.

This observation has opened new approaches for disease prevention.

approach *vt.* to begin to deal with

To approach a problem.

appropriate *adj.*

1. applicable, suitable

The study of laboratory animals is not always appropriate to human ageing.

This diet is appropriate for the patient's needs.

This treatment is not appropriate in pregnancy.

2. particular

These methods will be presented in appropriate chapters of this book.

Compare: applicable

appropriateness *n.* Appropriateness takes into consideration choices or decisions made in planning to see if they really were the best under the circumstances (WHO 1).

approval *n.* a formal agreement

Ethical committee approval was obtained for the study.

approve *vt.* to agree officially (to)

The drug has been approved in Britain.

approximately *adv.* about

Note: **about** is simpler and shorter.

apt *adj.* having a tendency

These haemorrhages /are apt to be/tend to be/are usually/ small.

Toxic reactions are apt to develop with impaired renal function.

arbiter *n.* a criterion

The histological picture was the final arbiter of diagnosis.

Compare: criterion

architecture *n.* structure

Histological studies showed disorganization of architecture indicating previous inflammation.

The tubular architecture was preserved in the operation.

To disrupt, disturb surface /architecture/features/ of a cell.

area *n.*

1. (the extent of) a body surface or functional region

The eruptions may appear on sun-exposed areas of the skin.

In a body area, on an area of the skin.

2. a geographical region

Patients from the Manchester area.

arguably *adv.* it may be argued that

Arguably, this symptom was a consequence of severe hyperglycaemia.

argue *vt.* to propose with reasons

/It might be argued that/arguably/ risk factors for retinopathy may be obscured if they also increase the risk of early death.

n. argument

arise (from) *vi.* to originate (from)

The inferior mesenteric artery arises from the aorta.

This deficiency may arise in adult life.

Cancer arising from the pancreas.

arm *n.* a subgroup of study subjects

A concurrent, untreated control arm.

The transplant group included four patients in the acyclovir arm and six in the placebo arm.

Compare: a leg of a study

armamentarium *n.* equipment and methods

This drug deserves a place in the psychiatrist's armamentarium of drugs for the treatment of depression.

arouse *vt.* give rise to

Stimuli arouse pain.

array *n.* group

An array of disorders.

arrest *n.* the sudden stopping of motion, progress or function

Cardiac arrest = the sudden cessation of arterial pulsation and heart sounds, with loss of consciousness.

Note: cardiac failure = cardiac insufficiency

arrest *vt.* to stop, inhibit (a process of progress)

Corticosteroids arrested the inflammation.

artefact (often AE:) **artifact** *n.* an unwanted factor that can produce false results in a study

These findings were an artefact resulting from the use of old sera.

artefactual, artifactual *adj.* pertaining to an artefact

Artefactual hyperkalaemia may be seen when potassium is measured in the serum of patients with thrombocytosis due to the release of potassium from platelets during clotting. The plasma potassium level is normal.

artificial *adj.* not natural, man-made

Artificial delay of the menopause.

Artificial kidney, respiration.

Artificial teeth = usually called dentures.

as *adv.* when considered from a specific point of view

She had normal renal function as assessed by creatinine clearance.

as *prep.*

1. in the state or condition

He was diagnosed as suffering from depression.

2. in the form of

This drug is available as tablets.

as *pron.* and so

Cytotoxic drugs may precipitate gout, as may allupurinol treatment.

ascending *adj.* rising

The ascending colon.

Opposite: descending

ascertain *vt.* to determine

To /ascertain/determine/ the effectiveness of a treatment.

ascribe to *vt.* to attribute to

We ascribed his epileptic seizures to acquired factors.

assay *vt.* to analyse by physical or biochemical methods

Serum samples were assayed by gas liquid chromatography.
The incubation mixture was assayed for conversion products
by electrophoresis.

adj. assayable

assay *n.* a determination or analysis

An immunofluorescence assay using monoclonal antibodies.

Clotting time assay.

Radioimmunoassays for progesterone.

To carry out an assay on a sample.

Urinary drug assay from samples.

assess *vt.* to determine, estimate, evaluate, examine

Each specimen was assessed for dysplasia and atrophy. A
score of 0–6 was used.

Patients may assess their symptoms themselves (= self-assess-
ment).

adj. assessable

assessment *n.* evaluation, estimation

To make an assessment of results.

Compare: appraisal

assign *vt.* to allot

To assign patients to a category, group.

Compare: allocate

assignment *n.* allotment

The random assignment of patients to groups.

assist *vt.* to help

Assisted ventilation.

The drug may /assist/plainly: help/ in reducing surgical bleeding.

associated with *adj.* connected with

Australian antigen is associated with one type of hepatitis.

Depressive states may be associated with antihypertensive
drugs.

This method is associated with recognizable hazards.

Strongly ⟷ weakly associated.

Verbal phrases referring to association: be associated with, be
connected to, be coupled with, be linked to; be contingent on,
be dependent on.

association *n.* the state of being associated; a connection

An inverse statistical /association/correlation/ has been found
between the risk of cancer and serum retinol concentrations.

A strong association between bird-keeping and this disease
may exist.

Chest pain and dysphagia occurred in close association.

assuage *vt.* to lessen, relieve

To assuage an alcoholic's craving for alcohol.

assume *vt.*

1. to suppose

We assumed that the patient had contracted the disease abroad.

Compare: presume

2. to take for oneself

The patient assumed the supine position.

assumption *n.* something that is taken for granted without proof

This investigation started on the assumption that food taken on a completely empty stomach is more likely to reach the areas usually affected by Crohn's disease.

asymptomatic *adj.* symptom-free

An asymptomatic patient.

asynchronous *adj.* not happening at the same time

pulsations asynchronous with carotid pulse.

at *prep.*

1. in connection with a procedure

Diagnosis was made at laparotomy.

2. under a certain condition

At a certain temperature.

3. using a certain rate

At a high concentration, frequency, intensity.

Whole blood was centrifuged at 1000 *g* for 10 minutes.

4. at a certain time (of observation)

At eight hours high drug concentrations were still present.

attach *vi. vt.* to fasten, join, connect

Hookworms attach by their mouths to the mucosa of the intestine.

attachment *n.*

1. the act of attaching

The attachment of monocytes to endothelial cells.

2. the point where something attaches

Bony outgrowth at the muscle attachment.

attack *n.* an episode of illness, usually acute

An attack of angina, asthma, back pain, claustrophobia.

A paroxysmal attack.

Petit mal attacks = petit mal seizures (in epilepsy).

Recurrent attacks of sleep.

The attack rate of an infection in a population.

To avert an attack.

Compare: bout, episode, fit, seizure

attain *vt.* to achieve, accomplish

To attain a goal.

n. attainment

attempt *n.* an effort made to do something

Attempts at activation of deficient intracellular enzymes.

Every possible attempt should be made to control these episodes.

There has been very little attempt to use this method for measuring antibodies.

In an attempt to = briefly: (in order) to:

Antibiotics have been used (in an attempt) to prevent viral disease complications.

attempt *vt.* to try to do something

Our study attempted to identify the location of this factor.

Parathyroidectomy was attempted in this patient.

attend *v.*

1. *vi.* to present for treatment

They attended the clinic at three-monthly intervals for urine culture

Compare: visit

2. *vt.* to be attended by = to be accompanied by

These disease states are attended by impaired renal potassium excretion.

3. *vi.* to treat a patient

To attend (on) a patient.

The attending physician (= the physician primarily in charge of or attending to a patient).

attendance *n.* a visit to a doctor or hospital

Her attendances were related to obesity.

The patients were questioned at each attendance at the outpatient clinic.

Their clinic attendance rate was poor.

Compare: consultation, visit

attendant *adj.* accompanying

Brain surgery and its attendant hazards.

attender *n.* one who attends

They were regular (⟷ poor) clinic attenders.

attention *n.*

1. full thought and consideration

Attention has been /concentrated/focused/ on the fibrotic features of systemic sclerosis.

The author drew attention to this important phenomenon.

This phenomenon has recently received considerable attention.

2. treatment, care

Expert attention was available.

He came under medical attention for hypertension. (= He presented with hypertension).

He sought medical attention at our hospital.

This condition requires scrupulous attention to foot hygiene.

This symptom brought the child to our attention.

This symptom requires immediate attention.

attenuate *vi. vt.* to make or become weak

Noise may be /attenuated/abated/ by wearing ear protectors.

Women may have the disorder in an attenuated form.

An attenuated vaccine, virus

n. attenuation

attractive *adj.* arousing interest, very tempting

Potassium phosphate is an attractive alternative parenteral preparation for this purpose.

attraction *n.* an interesting property

These animal models have obvious attractions.

attributable *adj.* able to be attributed

The high incidence of serious toxicity in our series may have been attributable to the high doses.

attribute to *vt.* to consider as being the result of

To attribute symptoms to a disease.

Compare: ascribe to, assign to

n. attribution

atypical *adj.* not conformable to the type

These symptoms were atypical for diabetes.

augment *vi. vt.* to add, increase, enlarge

To augment mitochondrial function.

To augment spontaneous labour.

n. augmentation

auscultate *vt.* to listen to and interpret body sounds

To auscultate lung bases for rales.

auscultation *n.* the diagnostic technique of listening

Auscultation by means of a stethoscope.

author *n.* the writer of a medical paper, a research worker

Many authors still fail to distinguish clearly between these more favourable forms of cancer of the pancreas.

v. author

authority *n.* an expert on a subject, a person or a publication mentioned as the source of certain information

Most authorities recommend caution in prescribing corticosteroid treatment in rheumatoid arthritis.

Most authorities advise, agree, believe, disagree that . . .

automotive *adj.* pertaining to automobiles (mainly AE)

These patients should not operate automotive equipment.

autonomous *adj.* independent, not secondary
    An autonomous tumour.
autopsy *n.* a post-mortem examination
    To examine an organ at autopsy.
    To verify by autopsy.
    Compare: necropsy, post-mortem examination
available *adj.*
    1. commercially obtainable
    Flavoured protein supplements are available.
    2. existing, at hand
    An emergency tray should be immediately available for these
    cases.
    The most convenient techniques currently available for this
    purpose.
    These values were not available in 10 patients.
    n. availability
avenue *n.* a means of access, route
    The plastic in-dwelling cannula /offers/provides/ a secure and
    reliable avenue for infusion.
average *vt.*
    1. To calculate the average of
    The six most recent blood glucose values were averaged as an
    index of glycaemic control.
    2. to have a mean value of
    The volume of the resting gastric juice averages about 50 ml.
average *n.* The *average* or *mean* most frequently employed in
    demography is the *arithmetic average* or *arithmetic mean* which
    consists of the sum of a number of quantities divided by their
    number (WHO 1).
    Their values were above ⟵⟶ below average.
    They smoked an average of more than 20 cigarettes daily.
    Compare: mean, median
    On average, they were three months older than the other
    children.
avert *vt.* to prevent
    To avert an attack, a disease.
    Vigorous sports tend to avert coronary heart disease.
avidity *adj.* greed
    The kidney's avidity for sodium.
    adj. avid
    Compare: affinity, predilection
avoid *vt.* to keep away from
    This surgical method avoids the major renal vessels.
avoidance *n.* the act of avoiding

Avoidance of cigarette smoking helps to avoid heart disease.

await *vt.* to wait for

Confirmation of these reports awaits more experience with the drug.

Routine clinical use of this new technique must await further study.

They were awaiting operation.

This finding awaits confirmation.

awake *adj.* not sleeping

Patients in the awake state.

The measurements were made in awake subjects.

awaken *vt.* to arouse from sleep

The pain of gastric ulcer may awaken the patient (from sleep) at night.

awakening *n.* the act of waking from sleep

Insomnia is associated with frequent awakenings from sleep and early awakenings.

aware *adj.* having knowledge

We /are aware of/plainly: know of/ other similar reports.

Compare: know, knowledge

awareness *n.*

1. knowledge

In recent years there has been a growing awareness that this method may be valuable in malignant bone diseases.

Prevention of adverse reactions requires awareness of the potential reactions.

The method has /broadened/heightened/ our /awareness/ plainly: knowledge/ of the role of macrophages in this disease.

2. consciousness

Episodes of altered awareness.

Distortions of spatial awareness.

B

baby *n.* an infant

A well-baby clinic.

bactericidal *adj.* destroying bacteria

The drug is bactericidal /for/to/ *Pneumococcus*.

balance *n.* a state of equilibrium

In parkinsonism the balance between dopamine and acetyl-choline is disturbed in the direction of cholinergic dominance.

To cause a negative nitrogen balance.

To maintain fluid balance.

To restore fluid and electrolyte balance.

Synonym: equilibrium

Opposite: imbalance

bank *n.* a depot of human material or tissues

A human-milk bank was established to serve the neonatal intensive care unit.

Blood, bone, eye, human milk, skin bank.

Compare: pool

bank *vt.* to store in a bank

Banked human blood.

barrier *n.* something that prevents or obstructs access, passage or progress

Amniotic fluid /acts as/is/ a barrier against mechanical shocks.

Heroin freely /crosses/passes/ the placental barrier.

Passage across a barrier.

The female urethra is an inefficient barrier to bacteria.

basal *adj.* serving as or forming the base

Basal levels of atriopeptin exist in the circulation, suggesting that it is released continuously at low levels. Increases can be elicited by high-salt diets.

Basal 24-hour urine samples were obtained.

base *vt.* to use as a basis

To base an argument on evidence.

based *v. part.*

Note: **based** is often used wrongly: – based on our data, we recommend this drug for hypertension.

Correct: on the basis of our data we recommend . . .

Correct: computerized measurements of blood pressure (which are) based on ultrasound

baseline (data, etc) *n.* data, etc. reflecting the state of affairs at the beginning of a programme or a programme phase, which serve as a point from which subsequent changes can be measured (WHO 1).

Before the study began, baseline fasting blood samples were obtained.

Scans were taken before treatment to provide a baseline for sequential assessment of regression of the tumour.

The baseline characteristics of the subjects were those at entry into the study.

basis *n.* something on which something else is established

Further studies will provide a sound basis for the understanding of this phenomenon.

The diagnosis was made on the basis of laboratory tests.

The psychological basis of anorexia.

To explain a phenomenon on the basis that . . .

She was treated on an outpatient basis = . . . as an outpatient.

batch *n.* a number or quantity occurring at the same time

A batch of antibodies, laboratory analyses.

A batch of tablets (the quantity produced at one operation of machinery).

battery *n.* a set or a series

A battery of measurements.

A battery of tests = a package of tests.

A diagnostic battery = a set of diagnostic procedures.

Compare: a panel, a programme of investigations

bear out *vt.* to confirm, to support

The results of our study do not bear out the views of other workers.

bearing *n.* relevance

These findings had an important bearing on the diagnosis.

become *vi.* to come to be

The ulcer became infected by streptococci.

Compare: the ulcer was infected by streptococci; *was* refers to a state, whereas *became* refers to transition to that state.

bed *n.* A *hospital bed* is one maintained for continuous (24-hour) use by inpatients (WHO 1)

They were in medical beds or surgical beds.

To allow a patient to sit out of bed.

To be confined to bed; confinement to bed.

To treat a patient on a plaster bed.

bed day *n.* a unit for the calculation of the use of hospital beds

The number of bed days used by this disease last year was high.

bed rest *n.* recovery and relaxation in bed

Bed rest is imperative, required for these patients.

His motor weakness resolved on bed rest.

To place/keep a patient on complete bed rest.

bedridden *adj.* confined to bed

To become bedridden.

Opposite: ambulatory

Compare: recumbent

bedside *n.* pertaining to procedures done at the side of the patient's bed

Biopsy at the bedside.

Diagnosis at the bedside = bedside diagnosis (as opposed to laboratory diagnosis).

Percutaneous needle biopsy is a simple bedside procedure.

The bedside availability of blood gas analysis.

bedtime *n.* the time of going to bed

The capsules were taken at bedtime.

Compare: meal (time)

begin *vt. vi* to start

To begin treatment.

behaviour (BE), **behavior** (AE) *n.* the activity of an organism, especially activity that can be observed

The accepted norms of sexual behaviour.

The appearance and behaviour of cancer cells are distinctive.

adj. behavioural (BE), behavioral (AE)

beneficial *adj.* producing a good result

A beneficial treatment.

Breathing exercises may be beneficial in asthma.

Opposite: detrimental

Compare: advantageous, helpful, useful

benefit *n.* good effect

He derived benefit from the treatment.

No benefit could be ascribed to the treatment.

The drug /brings/carries/gives/provides/ benefit in the treatment of angina.

The new method offers /benefits/advantages/ over the traditional treatment.

The treatment is /of benefit/plainly: useful/ in this disease.

This treatment is used to the great benefit of patients with angina.

A risk-versus-benefit analysis.

Compare: gain, helpfulness

benefit *vi. vt.*

1. *vt.* to improve, help

The treatment benefited patients with angina.

2. vi. to gain

These men benefited most from the treatment.

benign *adj.* not threatening to life or health

A benign tumour does not invade adjacent tissues or metastasize.

The generally /benign/favourable/good/ prognosis of mitral valve prolapse.

bias *n.* a latent influence that disturbs a statistical analysis

To avoid a bias in the selection of patients for a study (= selection bias).

The lack of male control subjects was a possible source of bias in this study.

bias *vt.* to cause deviation from a true value

The results of the study were biased by differences in the ages of the subjects.

bind *vi. vt.* to (cause to) become attached to

These antibodies bind to different areas of the epithelium.

These antibodies bind with hapten isomers.

A highly bound drug, a strongly bound drug.

binding *n.* the act or process of fastening

Strong ⟷ weak binding with antibody.

Total iron-binding capacity.

biopsy *n.* examination of tissue from a living body

To /carry out/do/ biopsy /in/on/ a patient, in an organ.

A renal biopsy was done.

To take a biopsy specimen.

Granulomas were found /at/on/ biopsy.

He underwent liver biopsy.

biopsy *vt.* to do biopsy

We biopsied the liver.

birth *n.* the act, fact or time of being born; parturition

At birth, the serum albumin is low.

Live birth ⟷ stillbirth.

She gave birth to a healthy child.

These women achieved a live birth.

Compare: delivery

bizarre *adj.* highly unusual (of appearance)

Bizarre behaviour, the bizarre shape of cells; bizarre cells.

bleed *vi.* to emit blood

A bleeding ulcer.

blind *adj.*

1. unable to see

The patient was blind in one eye.

2. without knowledge of certain facts (in a clinical trial)

A (double-) blind drug trial.

The nurses were /blind/blinded/ to the type of tablet used.
3. with only one opening
The caecum is a blind sac.

blind *vt.* to withhold information from test operators or subjects
The investigators were blinded to the identity of patients and controls.

block *vt.*
1. to obstruct, close, stop a channel or passage
The coronary arteries become blocked by atheroma and thrombosis.
Compare: obstruct
2. to suppress a response
His hypersensitivity reaction was blocked by sodium cromoglycate.

blockade *n.* the obstruction of a passage or process
The drug exerts selective blockade on receptors in specific tissues.

blockage *n.* an obstruction, the state of being blocked
Complete blockage of the oesophagus.

blood *n.* the red liquid which flows through the body
Banked blood, whole blood.
Blood was taken for laboratory tests.
Glucose concentrations in the blood.

blood-borne *adj.* carried in the blood
Tuberculosis of the adrenal gland is a blood-borne disease.

blood count *n.* the determination of blood cell numbers in a sample
To /do/carry out/take/ a blood count.
We did a blood count: erythrocyte count, leucocyte count, platelet count.

blood sample *n.* a blood specimen
Blood samples were collected by venepuncture from the subjects.

bloodstream *n.* the blood in the circulatory system
Infection may spread into the bloodstream.

blunt *vt.* to weaken (an effect)
The effects of the hormone were blunted by vitamin D deficiency.

body *n.*
1. a physical structure
The human body.
The pineal body = the pineal gland.
2. the main part of an organ
The body of the stomach.

bolus *n.* a round mass of food (to be) swallowed or a drug mass

Food is formed into a bolus by the action of the tongue and cheeks.

They were given bolus injections of the contrast medium.

bony *adj.* referring to bone

Bony changes such as demineralization.

Bony involvement.

boost *vt.* to increase

To boost the effect of a drug.

booster *n.* a substance or an effect prolonging a person's immunity to an infection

a booster dose of vaccine.

born *adj.* brought into existence by birth

Children born to mothers with rubella.

Compare: congenital, inborn, native

borne *adj.* transmitted

An air-borne, food-borne, insect-borne, water-borne infection

bound *adj.* held in a chemical combination

The zinc was firmly bound to globulins.

Opposites: free, unbound

bout *n.* an episode (of pain or fever)

Recurrent bouts of abdominal pain, nausea, nocturnal fever.

bowel *n.* intestine, the part of the alimentary canal beyond the stomach

The small/large bowel = the small/large intestine.

breakdown *n.*

1. decomposition

Breakdown products of drugs.

2. a sudden weakening or failure of physical or mental functions; collapse

A mental breakdown, a nervous breakdown.

3. division by types or into smaller groups; analysis

The breakdown of cases by the duration of treatment.

break down *v.*

1. to break into smaller units

Bile salts break down fats into smaller globules.

2. to analyse

To break down a report.

breathlessness *n.* the condition of gasping for air

She complained of breathlessness on slight exertion.

brief *adj.* short

Brief episodes of unconsciousness.

adv. briefly = in short

bring on *vt.* to cause to appear

The symptoms were brought on by exercise.

brisk *adj.* vigorous, intensive

Brisk diuresis, haemorrhage, reflexes.

brittle *adj.* (of diabetic patients:) unstable

A brittle diabetic = one who shows great oscillation between high and low blood glucose concentrations.

build-up *n.* a gradual increase

A build-up in the adrenal gland of androgens.

Compare: accumulation

build up *vi. vt.* to (cause to) increase gradually

Dosage was built up gradually.

Compare: titration

burden *n.*

1. a load, a large amount

Excessive fat is a burden to the heart.

The burden of ill heath.

The iron /burden/overload/ in patients requiring long-term transfusions.

The total known disease burden in the population.

2. a psychological problem

The burden imposed by ileostomy.

by *prep.*

1. by means of, by the use of

Diagnosis is (made) by scratch or intradermal test.

The drug was administered by an oral feeding tube.

The drug was given by intraperitoneal injection.

They were investigated by oesophagoscopy.

2. according to, on the basis of

They were classified by clinical and biochemical findings into four groups.

She was found seronegative by single radial haemolysis.

To judge by, identify by.

3. denoting degree, rate, etc.

The risk of coronary heart disease was reduced by 20%.

bypass *n.* a means of redirecting blood flow

A coronary bypass operation.

bypass *vi. vt.* to go around, avoid

Ammonia from the gastrointestinal tract bypasses the liver in severe hepatic decompensation.

C

cadaver *n.* a dead human body

A cadaver kidney = a cadaveric kidney.

They received kidneys from cadaver donors.

calculate *vt.* to count

To calculate cell numbers.

n. calculations

call *n.* duty

The consultant on /call/duty.

To be on surgical call.

Compare: duty

call for *vt.* to require

Agranulocytosis calls for an immediate change in treatment.

candidate *n.* a patient regarded as suitable for a treatment

They were (prospective, qualified, suitable) candidates for this treatment.

Compare: eligible

capable *adj.* able to carry out

Macrophages are not capable of phagocytosis.

This protein is capable of inhibiting endothelial replication in culture.

n. capability

capacity *n.* ability

The increased bone resorption exceeded the kidney's capacity to excrete calcium.

The liver has a remarkable capacity /for regeneration/ to regenerate/ after injury.

care *n.*

1. medical attention

Health care goes wider than medical care to embrace nursing care, dental care and many associated forms of care (WHO 1).

Intensive, maternity, medical, supportive, wound care.

To come under medical care.

To provide care for a patient.

2. caution

Great care was taken not to perforate the wall of the trachea.

*adj.*careful

care for *vi.* to treat

The hospital units caring for these patients.

carriage *n.*

1. transport

The carriage of oxygen by erythrocytes.

2. the act of carrying a disease, usually without clinical symptoms

In this disease carriage declines with age.

Families with one member suffering from pneumococcal disease have a high carriage rate.

carrier *n.*

1. a person or an organism that transmits disease from one host to another (without himself or itself suffering from the disease)

An asymptomatic carrier; a long-term, persistent carrier.

A persistent carrier state.

A reservoir of human carriers.

2. a carrier for a drug

The combination of nitroglycerine with a carrier from which it is slowly released.

Compare: vehicle.

carry *vt.*

1. to transport

Sensory fibres carry impulses to the brain.

The blood carries oxygen.

2. to harbour, transmit, and spread a disease

To carry a disease.

3. to be associated with

This maternal disease carries many /dangers/hazards/risks/ to the fetus.

carry out *vt.* to do

To carry out an analysis, a diagnosis, an examination, an experiment, a follow-up, an operation, a procedure, research, a survey, a test, work.

carry-over *n.* transfer (of an effect)

Few drug trials test for period effect or drug interaction, although some avoid the possibility of carry-over of a drug from one period to the next by allowing a wash-out period between different treatments.

carry over *vi.* to remain

This effect seemed to carry over from the previous treatment period.

case *n.*

1. an instance of a disease

Most cases in infants were diagnosed immediately.

The case illustrated in Fig. 1 is of a person with asthma.

2. a person suffering from a disease

Many consider the use of *case* instead of *patient* as inaccurate or unethical in scientific writing.

case-control *n.* a case-control study = a study of two groups of subjects – one with the disease (cases) and the other serving as controls

case-finding *n.* that form of *screening* of which the main object is to detect disease and bring patients to treatment, in contrast to *epidemiological surveys* (WHO 1).

case history *n.* a record of a patient's medical background, history
See: history

catch *vt.* to detect
The disease can be treated effectively if /caught/usually: diagnosed/ early.

catchment area *n.* an area which is served by a particular treatment unit
This colposcopy clinic serves a large catchment area.

categorize, categorise *vt.* to put into a category
They were categorized as having 'possible heart disease'.
Compare: classify

category *n.* a division in a classification system
The patients fell into the high-risk category.
To assign a patient to a category.

causal *adj.* acting as or being a cause, showing a relationship
A causal agent.
A causal /link/relationship/ between two conditions.

causally *adv.* from the causal point of view
Osteoporosis is causally related to the loss of ovarian function.

causation *n.* the act or process of causing
An infectious agent may be involved in the causation of cervical cancer.

causative *adj.* producing an effect
A causative agent, organism.
To /have/play/ a causative role in a disease.

cause *n.* the thing, event, state or action that produces an effect
An underlying cause, the immediate cause.
An ulcer was the cause of the abdominal pain.
No cause was found for the abdominal pain.
To avoid, eliminate/establish/identify/, remove, treat the cause of a disease
These signs gave cause for concern.

cause *vt.* to bring about
Ectopic cilia may cause corneal ulceration.
Papaverine /causes relaxation of/relaxes/ smooth muscle.
Other verbal constructions expressing causation: be ascribable to, be attributable to, be due to, be responsible for; give rise to, induce, lead to, produce

caution *n.* care, prudence

Use this drug with caution in patients with peptic ulcer.

Use caution in giving the drug.

This procedure calls for judicious caution.

caution *vt.* to warn

They were cautioned about engaging in activities requiring mental alertness and motor coordination.

They were cautioned against operating cars and machinery.

cautionary *adj.* intended to warn

With this drug, a cautionary note is necessary, as with any new drug.

cavity *n.*

1. hollow space in the body, normal or pathological

In pulmonary tuberculosis, foci of infection tend to progress and form new cavities.

The abdominal cavity, the cranial cavity.

2. the lesion or area of a tooth destroyed by caries

Caries results in the erosion of the enamel and dentine of the teeth leading to the formation of cavities.

cease *vi. vt.* to (cause to) come to an end

He ceased to breathe = His breathing ceased.

n. cessation

ceiling *n.* an upper limit

The ceiling of morphine's analgesic effect is very high.

central *adj.*

1. most important

These procedures are central to the management of the disease.

2. pertaining to the central nervous system

Central neurological lesions.

Opposite: peripheral

centre (BE), **center** (AE)

1. the most important part of a system

A thermoregulatory centre in the hypothalamus controls the temperature of the body.

2. a central institution (often with a large catchment area)

A cardiac centre with regional responsibility.

Clinical, health, referral, research, special(ist), treatment centre.

certify *vt.* to declare

He was certified as having died of tuberculosis.

cessation *n.* a temporary or final ceasing; discontinuation

The cessation of arterial pulsation.

The cessation of cigarette smoking.

The /cessation/usually: discontinuation/ of the drug is followed by the return of granulocytes to normal.

A smoking-cessation clinic.

v. cease

challenge *vt.* to administer a substance to evoke a response in an individual

challenge *n.* a test of immunity or susceptibility

A gluten challenge in coeliac disease.

Confirmation of diagnosis by challenge with the suspected antigen.

These cells may confer protection against viral challenge.

Compare: tolerance (test)

change *n.* the act or result of changing

A noticeable change occurred in the patient.

Other nouns expressing change:

abatement, decline, diminution, drop, elevation, increase ⟷ decrease, increment, reduction, rise ⟷ fall

Adjectives collocating with these nouns:

appreciable, considerable, dramatic, drastic, great, marked, mild, moderate, severe, sharp, slight, steady

change *vi. vt.* to (cause to) become different

He changed from this drug to penicillin.

He was changed to penicillin.

Treatment A was changed to treatment B.

Other verbs expressing change:

abate, aggravate ⟷ alleviate, allay, ameliorate ⟷ deteriorate, amplify, assuage, attenuate, augment, boost, compound, decline, diminish, drop, increase ⟷ decrease, lessen, reduce, rise ⟷ fall

Adverbs collocating with these verbs:

appreciably, considerably, dramatically, drastically, greatly, markedly, mildly, moderately, severely, sharply, slightly, steadily.

changeover *n.* switch

A changeover from one drug to another.

character *n.* nature, qualities

We studied the character of jerks in epileptic myoclonus.

characterize, characterise *vt.*

1. to describe the character of

To characterize a virus.

2. to be typical of

Chronic proctitis is characterized by fibrosis of the rectal wall.

characteristic *adj.* typical

A characteristic feature of this aneurysm is that it bulges

outwards from the ventricular wall = characteristically, this aneurysm bulges . . .

characteristic *n.* a typical feature

Hypertension is one of the main characteristics of this disease.

Compare: hallmark

charge *n.* responsibility

A doctor is in charge of his patients.

child-bearing *adj.* bringing forth children

Women /of child-bearing age/ in their child-bearing years.

chill *n.* (often plural:) a sensation of coldness followed by shivering

Shaking chills are seen in many bacterial infections.

choice *n.*

1. the act of choosing

The choice of a drug for treatment.

2. the best

In these patients surgery is the treatment of choice.

Tetracyclines are not the drug of choice in the treatment of this infection.

chronic disease, illness *n.* an impairment of bodily structure and/or function that necessitates a modification of the patient's normal life, and has persisted or may be expected to persist over an extended period of time (WHO 1).

Chronic treatment = usually: long-term treatment.

Compare: prolonged, long-term; acute

chronicity *n.* the quality of being chronic

The chronicity of a disease.

circadian *adj.* of a process occurring regularly at 24-hour intervals

The circadian pattern of sodium excretion.

The circadian rhythm of hormone secretion.

circularize, circularise *vt.* to send a letter to many people

All students known to have a history of hay fever were circularized.

n. circularization, circularisation

circulate *vi.* to move about

This peptide circulates in the blood.

circulation *n.* flow of fluid in the body, often = blood circulation

Vitamin A is released into the circulation as retinol.

circulatory *adj.* relating to (blood) circulation

Circulatory collapse, compromised circulatory states.

circumstance *n.* (usually plural:) a condition influencing an event or a person

Laparotomy was carried out /in/under/ difficult circumstances.

The social circumstances of a patient.

cite *vt.* to refer to (in published papers)

Cachexia has been cited as the most common cause of death in patients with cancer.

n. citation

clammy *adj.* moist, unpleasantly sticky

His skin was cold and clammy.

clarification *n.* the act of making clearer

Further studies are needed for clarification of this problem.

clarify *vt.* to make clear

How antibody formation is induced remains to be clarified.

classic, classical *adj.* belonging to an established set of scientific standards or methods

The classical, conventional method ←——→ the new method.

The classic(al) symptoms of a disease.

classification *n.* the act or result of classifying

To base a classification on certain factors.

classify *vt.* to arrange in classes

The cases were classified by biochemical findings.

These drugs are classified into three groups.

clean *vt.* to remove dirt

Burned areas should be cleaned with soap and water.

cleanse *vt.* to remove dirt

The wounds were cleansed with hydrogen peroxide.

clear *adj.*

1. free from doubt

It was clear that the deficiency was due to this factor.

This is clear from many reports.

Clear evidence emerged.

Compare: unequivocal

2. free from disease

A clear skin = skin without rash

The lung fields were clear.

clear *vi. vt.*

1. *vt.* to make clear, open, remove obstruction

To clear a microscopical specimen = to remove its cloudiness by a clearing agent or clearer.

To clear the airways by suction.

2. *vt.* to eliminate from the bloodstream

Indium is cleared through the liver.

3. *vi.* to heal

The rash cleared without scarring.

clearance *n.*

1. disappearance

The clearance of all obvious deposits of tumour.

2. elimination

The clearance of bacterial infections by antibiotics.

The clearance of carbon dioxide by the lungs.

clearing *n.* disappearance

The clearing and continued remission of psoriasis.

The clearing of warts was defined as the disappearance of all treated warts in a patient.

cleavage *n.* (a) division or split

The activation of the components of the complement system involves enzymatic cleavage of each component into two fragments.

v. cleave

clinic *n.* a unit for diagnosis and treatment

They were managed in hospital clinics.

clinical *adj.* pertaining to the clinic or to the bedside; actual observation and treatment of patients as opposed to theoretical or basic medical science; observable by clinical methods.

clinical can sometimes be omitted without affecting the clarity of the expression.

Compare: experimental(ly induced); theoretical

Clinical studies ⟷ research studies, pathological or laboratory findings.

clinical course *n.*

The drug shortens the clinical course of this disease.

clinical death *n.* death as assessed by clinical methods

clinical finding *n.* a finding by clinical methods

clinical improvement *n.* improvement as assessed by clinical methods

These measures led to prompt clinical improvement.

clinical picture *n.* clinical signs and symptoms

The patient's clinical picture was characterized by pallor.

The two diseases produce a similar clinical picture.

clinical setting *n.* the relevant clinical circumstances

Each finding must be evaluated in the context of the overall clinical setting.

clinical sign *n.* a sign of a disease as seen in an ordinary medical examination

clinical status *n.* the patient's status as observed clinically

LATS responses should be correlated with the patient's clinical status.

clinical trial *n.* a study in which a drug or a procedure is assessed for the diagnosis, treatment or prophylaxis of a disease

clinically *adv.*

1. by clinical methods

A clinically diagnosed urinary tract infection.

2. from the clinical point of view
Clinically important bleeding

close *vt.* to bring the edges of a wound or incision together
To close an open wound surgically.

closure *n.*
1. the act of closing
The surgical closure of the front of the bladder.
2. a cap or seal of a container
Drugs in a bottle with a child-resistant closure.

clouded *adj.* confused
Clouded consciousness.

clue *n.* something that may lead to the solution of a problem
The laboratory studies gave clues /to/for/ diagnosis.

cluster *n.* a number of similar things occurring together
Leukaemia clusters have been reported around nuclear plants.

clustering *n.* occurrence together
Environmental factors may account for familial clustering of this disease.

coalesce *vi.* to unite
The papules coalesce /into/to form/ scaly patches.

coarse *adj.* rough
A coarse ⟷ fine tremor.

coated *adj.* covered with an enclosing layer
The aspirin tablets were enteric-coated.

coated *n.* a layer over a surface
A protein coat
v. coat

coauthor *n.* a research worker as a contributor to a report etc.
Brown and his coauthors
Compare: *et al.*

code *n.* a system of secret letters or digits used (often in clinical trials) instead of ordinary writing
The code was broken and the treatment group identified.
Note: the genetic code of DNA

coexist *vi.* to exist together
Shoulder pain and cervical spondylosis often coexist in the elderly.
n. coexistence
Compare: coincide

coexistent *adj.* existing together
Tuberculosis pericarditis and coexistent pulmonary tuberculosis.
Compare: concomitant, concurrent

cofactor *n.* a factor acting together with another

Infection with Epstein-Barr virus in association with environmental cofactors, possibly endemic malaria, has been proposed as having a critical role in the development of African Burkitt's lymphoma.

cohort *n.* A group of persons who experience a certain event in a specified period of time (WHO 1)

The original cohort was recruited to the study programme in 1980.

coincide *vi.*
1. to occur simultaneously
These assessments coincide with patients' outpatient appointments.
2. to be in agreement with
The clinical picture coincided with the results of laboratory tests.
adj. coincident.

coincidental *adj.* occurring at the same time
The patient had benign monoclonal gammopathy with a coincidental renal-cell carcinoma.

collaboration *n.* cooperation
To work in collaboration.
adj. collaborative

collapse *n.*
1. the complete failure of a system
Patients in cardiovascular collapse.
She suffered a nervous collapse.
2. the abnormal caving-in of the wall of an organ
The collapse of a lung in pneumothorax.

collapse *vi. vt.*
1. *vi.* to fall into a flattened, reduced mass
The lung had collapsed as a result of the bronchial obstruction.
2. *vi.* to fall down suddenly, often with loss of consciousness
The patient collapsed.
3. *vt.* to cause to fall down or cave in
The lung was collapsed as a therapeutic measure.

collect *vt.* to gather
Faecal samples were collected for three days /in/from/ patients.
n. collection

colonize, colonise *vt.* to establish a bacterial colony
Those treated with immunosuppressive drugs are likely to be colonized by unusual organisms such as *Candida*.
n. colonization, colonisation

colony *n.* a bacterial group of culture

A daughter, satellite colony.

coma *n.* a profound unconsciousness

She was admitted in (a) coma.

She went into (a) coma.

She died in (a) coma.

adj. comatose

combat *vt.* fight

To combat a disease, a condition.

n. combat

combination *n.* a product of combining

A combination tablet including frusemide and amiloride.

A drug may be given in combination with another drug, or singly.

Compare: alone

combine *vi. vt.* to (cause to) unite

An antibody combines with an antigen.

To combine a drug with another treatment.

commence *vt.* (more formal than:) to begin, to start

To commence treatment = to start treatment.

n. commencement = start

commensurately *adv.* coincidentally with in degree, extent, etc.

Efforts should be made to reduce the daily dose commensurately with evidence of improvement.

commercially *adv.* on the market

Commercially available bacterial preparations.

common *adj.* occurring frequently, usual

Hypovolaemia is common with prolonged use of thiazides.

adv. commonly

communicable *adj.* that can be transmitted

A communicable disease.

Compare: contagious, transmittable

communicability *n.* capacity for being communicated

The disease has a high rate of communicability.

communicate *vi. vt.*

1. to transmit

This disease is easily communicated.

Compare: spread, transmit

2. to be connected with

Most arteries communicate with other arteries.

communication *n.* exchange of facts and opinions

More concretely: article, letter, paper

A personal communication (as opposed to published work) = a letter or telephone call, etc.

community *n.* a group in face-to-face contact – having a basic harmony of interest and aspirations and bound by common values and objectives. It can be geographical, socio-economic, professional, etc. It can be small – a village, a factory; it can be large – up to a region (WHO 1).

Community care ←——→ hospital inpatient care, especially but not exclusively in the mental health field.

Hospital and community medicine.

These patients can live in the community under the care of general practitioners.

comparable *adj.* able to be compared (to, with), similar

All patients underwent comparable diagnostic procedures.

40 mg of the drug are comparable in analgesic effect to 10 mg of morphine.

The incidence of side-effects with placebo was comparable to that observed with active treatment.

comparability *n.* the quality or state of being comparable

The comparability of the results of two separate studies.

comparative *adj.*

1. of or involving comparison

Comparative anatomy, a comparative study.

2. used for comparison

The other patient group provided a useful comparative yardstick.

compare

1. *vi. vt.* to examine or assess one thing against another to show similarities and differences

A long-acting nitroglycerine preparation was compared /to/ against/ placebo.

The effects of the two drugs were compared in 20 patients (= in a comparative study).

The groups were compared for age, weight, parity and social class.

To compare to = to liken: The skull may be compared to a heavy ball on the end of a chain.

As/when/ compared with = briefly: than

We found a lower incidence of such arrhythmias in normal individuals /when compared with/simply: than in/ patients who had had a myocardial infarction.

2. to be comparable or equal

Drug X compares favourably with drug Y in analgesic potency.

comparison *n.* the act of comparing

A comparison between two drugs = a between-drug comparison.

A comparison of drug A and drug B for severity of pain.

In comparison with = when compared with = often: than.

compatible *adj.*

1. consistent with (the signs and symptoms of)

The adrenal biopsy specimen showed an interstitial lymphocytic infiltrate compatible with rejection.

2. able to coexist

The maximum degree of dehydration compatible with life is about 20%.

The mild form of the disease is compatible with long life.

3. suitable for simultaneous administration

Compatible ⟷ incompatible drugs.

compensate *vt.* to counterbalance, counteract undesirable effects

The healthy heart compensates for the reduction in cardiac rate by an increase in stroke volume.

Compare: make up (for)

compensatory *adj.* serving to compensate

In anoxia, the accumulation of carbon dioxide produces compensatory responses.

compete *vt.* to try to win in competition with something else

To compete for a binding site.

competence *n.* the ability of a part or a system to carry out its function

Cardiac, immune competence.

Opposite: incompetence

competent *adj.* able to perform a specific function

Competent valves.

Immunocompetent ⟷ immunosuppressed.

competition *n.* rivalry

Competition for a binding site on a molecule.

Strong ⟷ weak competition.

complain of *v.* to state the presence of symptoms

He complained of a headache.

complaint *n.* a symptom

Anorexia is a common complaint of patients with cancer.

The drug was associated with 2–6 complaints per patient.

Compare: ailment, disease, disorder, symptom

complete *adj.* full

Complete recovery is usual in this disease.

adv. completely

Opposite: incomplete

complete *vt.* to finish

The study was completed in four weeks.

completely *adv.* wholly, altogether

The disease attacks stopped completely.

completeness *n.* the state of being complete

The duration and completeness of remission induced by treatment.

completion *n.* the process or result of finishing

The completion of a study.

compliance *n.* adherence to instructions

Good ⟷ poor compliance with instructions, recommendations.

adj. compliant

Opposite: non-compliance

complicate *vt.* to add new developments to a disease

Pneumonia may complicate severe chickenpox.

The infection was complicated by aseptic meningitis.

complication *n.* a new disease or disorder arising during the course of another disease.

A ureteric fistula is a dreaded complication in the immuno-suppressed patient.

This disease is usually benign unless complications ensue.

They /experienced/encountered/simply: had/ complications.

comply *vi.* to act according to instructions

To comply well ⟷ poorly.

They complied with treatment instructions.

component *n.* part, ingredient

Cholesterol is the major component of deposits in the lining of arteries.

compose of *vt.* to make up

This membrane is composed of three layers.

n. composition

compound *vt.* to intensify by an added element

Multisystemic manifestations are usual in necrobacillosis and compound the diagnostic confusion.

The hypovolaemia was compounded when fluid was withheld.

Compare: aggravate; add to, increase

comprehension *n.* the act or process of grasping with the intellect

She had problems in comprehension at school.

compress *vt.* to push firmly and steadily in contact

Bed-sores arise when the skin is compressed against bone.

n. compression

comprise *vt.* to consist of, include

A course comprised six treatments = six treatments constituted a course.

Compare: contain, include

compromise *n.* weakness of function

Cardiac, renal compromise.

Compare: failure, insufficiency

compromised *adj.* inefficient, weakened, reduced

Acute streptococcal infections may invade tissue compromised by trauma.

Compromised cardiac output due to myocardial disease.

If the liver is diseased, lactic acid removal will be compromised.

Immunocompromised = immunologically weakened.

compute *vt.* to calculate

To compute the average age of a patient group.

computed *adj.* done by a computer

Computed tomographic scan.

computer *n.* an electronic machine for data processing

Data were stored in a computer.

The results were automatically recorded on computer files.

computerized, computerised *adj.* processed by means of a computer

Computerized death certificate registries.

Computerized/computed/ x-ray tomography.

conceivable *adj.* possible to think

It is conceivable that lack of exercise was a contributory factor to his disease.

conceive *vt.* to think of, consider to be

The author conceived this area in the distal tubule as a primary sensing element.

Compare: consider

concentrate *v.*

1. *vt.* to make less dilute

Bile becomes concentrated in the gall bladder.

The ability of the kidney to concentrate the urine.

Opposite: dilute

2. *vi.* to direct attention to

We concentrated on the mechanism by which acupuncture acts rather than its clinical effect on chronic pain.

Compare: focus

concentration *n.* the relative content of a component

A fall ⟵⟶ rise in a concentration.

The drug reached peak plasma concentrations at one hour.

They received oxygen /at/in/ high concentrations.

We /attained/obtained/ effective blood concentrations with oral doses of 80 mg/day.

Compare: content, level

concept *n.* a general idea, notion

This concept is not tenable, it can be disputed.

Compare: hypothesis, theory

concerned *adj.* taking part in, involved

Neutrophil granulocytes are concerned with combating bacterial infections.

Red cells are concerned in this process.

concert *n.* agreement

In concert with = in agreement, together.

conclude *vt.* to come to a conclusion

To conclude something /on the basis of/from/ a study.

Compare: infer

conclusion *n.*

1. end

At the /conclusion/completion/ of the study.

2. the outcome of (a study); inference

A firm, tentative, conclusion can be /made/drawn/reached// about /from/on/ these findings.

in conclusion = as the last thing (summarizing what has been said above)

/In conclusion/in summary/, the study has shown that the treatment is well tolerated.

conclusive *adj.* irrefutable

Conclusive evidence.

conclusively *adv.* in a conclusive manner

The survival benefit of postoperative radiation in this disease has been conclusively demonstrated.

concomitant *adj.* occurring together

Bacterial resistance is delayed by concomitant administration of a second drug.

Concomitant pathological conditions, findings.

Congenital rubella and concomitant growth-hormone deficiency.

Compare: concurrent, coexistent

n. concomitance

concurrent *adj.* occurring at the same time

The side-effects were abolished by stopping concurrent medication with benzhexol.

condition *n.*

1. conditions = circumstances

The test was carried out under standard conditions.

2. ailment, disease, illness, physical disability

A degenerative condition, such as arthritis.

3. state of health, fitness

Physical condition, mental condition.

He was in good physical condition.

His condition improved ⟵⟶ worsened.

conduct *vt.* to carry out

To conduct an enquiry, an examination, an experiment, an investigation, a procedure, research, a study, a survey, a test, a trial.

Compare: carry out, do, make

confer *vt.* to give

To /confer/plainly: have/ a benefit.

To /confer/plainly: carry/ a risk.

This factor may confer cytotoxicity on lymph node cells.

To /confer/give/provide/immunity, protection, against an infection

confine *vt.*

1. to restrict

This disease is confined to heavy smokers.

Patients confined by illness to bed, to a dwelling, to the house, to a wheelchair.

2. to keep in bed to give birth to a child

She was confined on the 18th and delivered on the 19th.

confinement *n.* the period of being confined (often for the delivery of a baby)

The trend is towards shorter hospital /confinements/stays.

Confinement to bed.

confirm *vt.* to give new supporting evidence

The diagnosis was confirmed /at/by/ laparotomy.

This study confirms that . . .

adj. confirmable

Compare: bear out, establish, validate

confirmation *n.* the act or result of confirming

To /obtain confirmation of/confirm/ a disease.

confirmative *adj.* serving to confirm

Confirmative diagnostic evidence.

confirmatory *adj.* confirmative

A confirmatory finding.

conflict *vi.* to be in disagreement

This finding conflicts with the results of previous studies.

Conflicting views have appeared in various reports about the value of this diagnostic sign.

conflict *n.* disagreement

A major conflict surrounds this usual treatment recommendation.

conformity *n.* agreement

In conformity with:

Our observations are in /conformity/usually: agreement/ with those of Hill *et al.*

confuse *vt.* to fail to tell the difference between two things

This disease is often confused with osteoarthritis.

n. confusion

Compare: mistake

congenital *adj.* present at birth

congenital disorders = those diseases that are substantially determined before or during birth and which are in principle recognizable in early life (WHO 1).

A congenital ⟷ acquired disease.

A congenital anomaly, malformation.

conjunction *n.* combination

Probenecid is not used in /conjunction/combination/ with penicillin in patients with renal impairment.

connection *n.* relation(ship)

The possible connection between repeated sunburns and skin cancer.

consciousness *n.* the state of being conscious

He lost ⟷ regained consciousness.

His level of consciousness deteriorated ⟷ improved.

Compare: awareness

consecutive *adj.* following one another without interruption

Two consecutive serum samples were positive for the antigen.

consensus *n.* a general agreement

Consensus favours this method in the treatment of the disease.

There is /consensus/general agreement/ on how this disease should be treated.

consent to *vi.* to agree to

They consented to participate in the trial with full knowledge of its content and implications.

They freely consented to the operation.

consent *n.* agreement

Informed consent = the patient's consent to take part in a medical experiment after the procedure has been explained to him and he has understood clearly the risk involved in it.

Their consent was obtained after a clear, thorough explanation of the programme, its goals, and its known risks.

They gave written consent to participate in the study in the full knowledge of the procedures to be undertaken.

Written parental consent.

consequence *n.* a result, effect

Pulmonary infarction is an infrequent consequence of pulmonary embolism.

Compare: complication, sequel

consequent *adj.*

1. resulting

An infection and the consequent symptoms.

2. consequent on = often simply: as a result of

This defect may be acquired consequent on uraemia.

consequently *adv.* as a result

This is a serious symptom and, consequently, it must be combated vigorously.

consider *vt.*

1. to think carefully about

They were considered for transfer to another hospital.

2. to judge, regard

He was considered to have Wilson's disease.

We consider this (to be/as/) a major problem.

Compare: regard as

considerable *adj.* worth consideration; great, high, large

Arteries carry blood at a considerable pressure.

Note: The word is sometimes unnecessary.

considerably *adv.* to a considerable extent, appreciably

His condition improved considerably.

Note: The word is sometimes unnecessary.

consideration *n.* = a fact that should be considered

A major consideration with any new drug is its side-effects.

To take into consideration = often simply: consider.

consist *vi.*

1. consist of = to be composed of

The heart consists of four chambers.

Compare: be made up of

2. consist in = to depend on

The treatment of this disease consists in the correction of the electrolyte disturbances.

consistent with *adj.*

1. in agreement with

Our results are consistent with their observations.

2. compatible

He presented with signs and symptoms consistent with the diagnosis of pulmonary embolism.

adj. inconsistent

n. consistency

Compare: compatible

constant *adj.*

1. unchanging, unchanged

A constant rate of infusion.

Their daily intake of fluid remained constant.

2. occurring all the time

This was a constant finding in our patients.

constantly *adv.* all the time

The eyes are never still: they constantly undergo minute oscillatory movements.

constellation *n.* a group, a set

A new constellation of symptoms was observed in this patient.

constituent *adj.* being one or several of the parts of a whole

Macrophages are the major constituent in fibrous plaques (= they are the predominant type of cell).

constitute *vt.* make up

High plasma cholesterol levels constitute a risk factor for coronary heart disease.

They constituted one half of the total patient population.

Compare: comprise

constitution *n.* physical nature or disposition

Bronchial asthma is found in individuals with an inherited allergic constitution.

constitutional *adj.* pertaining to constitution

Constitutional symptoms, such as fever, headache, malaise.

construct *vt.* to create (surgically)

A surgically constructed portacaval anastomosis.

n. construction

consult *vt.* to see a doctor for advice

To consult a physician /because of/for/ persistent headache.

Compare: see

consultation *n.* a meeting of two or more individuals who are seeking through the exchange of information to arrive at a decision (WHO 1).

Surgery consultation ⟷ domiciliary consultation.

contact *vt.* to come in touch with

To contact a doctor.

Compare: consult, seek (medical attention)

contact *n.* close association or physical union

An infection resulting from contact with monkeys.

The part of the skin that comes /in/into/ contact with this substance is affected.

To /be/lie/ in contact with.

To bring two things into contact.

contagion *n.* transmission of a disease

contagious *adj.* communicable

A contagious disease.

contain *vt.* to hold

The axilla contains a group of lymph nodes.

contaminate *v.* to make impure or bad; infect

The water had been contaminated by rats.

contamination *n.* the act or result of contaminating

The bandages gave protection against bacterial contamination.

contemplate *vt.* to consider carefully

Surgery was contemplated in this patient in whom medical treatment was no longer effective.

n. contemplation

content *n.* the amount or proportion of a component in a mixture

A low ⟷ high renal renin content.

Compare: concentration, level

context *n.* relevant circumstances

These clinical signs may be unreliable /in the context of/in/ severe head injury.

contingent *adj.* dependent on

The treatment of patients with bronchogenic carcinoma /is contingent on/usually: depends on/ accurate staging.

continuation *n.*

1. the act of continuing

The continuation of treatment.

2. something that continues

The axillary artery is the continuation of the subclavian artery.

continue *vt.* to carry on

To continue ⟷ /discontinue/stop/ a drug, a treatment.

continuous *adj.* going on without interruption

These women received continuous oestrogen treatment.

The rectum is /continuous with/a continuation of/ the sigmoid colon

adv. continuously

contract *vt.*

1. to make or become smaller, shorter, etc.

A muscle contracts ⟷ relaxes.

To contract ⟷ expand one's chest.

2. to acquire a disease

Man may /contract/acquire/ melioidosis by inhalation, but not directly from infected patients.

contradiction *n.* the action or result of contracting

The contraction ⟷ relaxation of a muscle.

The rhythmic contraction of the stomach in a hungry person.

The contraction of a disease.

contractile *adj.* that can contract

A contractile muscle.

contradict *vt.* to be in conflict or direct opposition with

This conclusion contradicts that reached by previous studies.

contradictory *adj.* serving to contradict

The results of these two studies are contradictory.

The views of these authors are divergent or even contradictory.

Compare: conflicting

contraindicate *vt.* to advise against the use of a particular drug or treatment; often used in the passive

The drug is strictly contraindicated in women of child-bearing age, in anuria.

There is no convincing evidence to contraindicate moderate-dose oestrogen treatment for the relief of these symptoms.

contraindication *n.* a sign, symptom or condition making the use of a drug inadvisable

A history of hypersensitivity to this drug is a contraindication /for/to/ its use.

contrary *adj.* wholly opposed

Our findings are contrary to the results of previous studies.

contrary *n.* the opposite

On the contrary = just the opposite.

The author does not advocate this method. On the contrary, he considers it too hazardous for clinical use.

Compare: on the other hand = it is, however, also true that . . . : We were the first to describe the mechanism. On the other hand, we misinterpreted its role.

to the contrary = exactly opposite:

The court decided that spermicides could be called teratogens despite the preponderance of medical evidence to the contrary.

contrast

1. *vi.* to show a difference when compared

These findings contrast with earlier findings.

2. *vt.* to compare two things so that their differences are made clear.

Brown contrasted his findings with ours.

contrast *n.* emphasis of difference by comparison of dissimilarities

These results are in clear, sharp, striking, contrast to those of previous studies.

In contrast /to/with/ patients with hypopituitarism, these patients may have increased plasma growth hormone levels.

A contrast medium.

contrasting *adj.* of opposite quality

Contrasting findings.

contribute to *vt.* to have a share in bringing about
    All these factors contributed to his hypertension.
    n. contribution
contributory to *adj.* helping to bring about
    Chemical analysis of the crystals was a contributory factor in
    the diagnosis of urinary calculi.
    Opposite: non-contributory
control *n.*
    1. governing or limitation
    Adequate, effective, sufficient, tight, control of poliomyelitis
    has been /achieved/attained/ in many areas.
    The infection /has been brought/is/ under control.
    This dosage of the drug seems to give adequate control of the
    disease.
    To achieve moderate, good ⟷ poor control of asthma,
    diabetes.
    To lose dietary control in a child.
    2. monitoring
    This intravenous drug should be given slowly under electro-
    cardiographic control.
    3. the standard of comparison in a study
    Age-matched, non-pregnant controls were used.
    Healthy children served as controls.
    Healthy, hospital, outpatient controls.
    The study group ⟷ the control group.
    Control diabetics.
    Control knees = intact knees (in a surgical trial).
    The control tissue was taken from sites 3–5 cm from the
    tumours.
control *vt.*
    1. to limit the progress or spread of a disease
    The attacks were inadequately controlled by the drug.
    2. to verify by conducting a parallel experiment
    Well-controlled studies in normal adult volunteers showed
    that the drug was well tolerated.
    3. to limit the effect of a factor
    The method of Mantel was used to control for age.
controllable *adj.* able to be controlled
    The bleeding /was controllable/could be controlled/ by
    heparin.
    Opposite: uncontrollable.
controversial *adj.* causing argument or disagreement
    The causative relationship between plasma lipid and coronary
    thrombosis is still controversial.

controversy *n.* a dispute, debate

There is controversy /about/over/ the optimal diet in this disease.

This current controversy remains unresolved.

This mechanism is /a subject of controversy/surrounded by controversy/controversial/.

This question has /produced/provoked/ controversy.

convention *n.* the accepted view, often without sufficient evidence or foundation

Current /convention/thinking/wisdom/ regards gall stones that appear radiolucent on oral cholecystography as being made up of cholesterol.

Compare: consensus

conventional *adj.* established in accepted practice, traditional

Conventional techniques as opposed to our new assay.

conversion *n.* a change

Conversion for something /to/into/ something.

The conversion of one substance to another.

convert *vt.* to change

Fatty acid cannot be converted /to/into/ glucose.

Superinfections may convert a benign disease into a serious one.

convey *vt.* carry

To convey nervous impulses.

Compare: carry

cooperation *n.* working together; help, support

This method requires no cooperation from the patient.

Compare: collaboration

cornerstone *n.* a thing of utmost importance, basis

Penicillin remains the cornerstone of the treatment of syphilis.

Compare: keystone, linchpin

correct *vt.*

1. to adjust a factor or a value to some standard condition or regimen

Faecal calcium and phosphorus values were corrected for barium sulphate which was used as a marker.

Compare: adjust

2. to treat or cure

To correct a defect.

She was given a preparation to correct her anaemia.

Compare: rectify

correctable, correctible *adj.* that must or can be corrected

An urgently correctable lesion.

Surgically correctable conditions.

correction *n.*

    1. adjustment

    The correction of test values for age and sex.

    Compare: adjustment

    2. treatment

    The correction of hypocalcaemia with vitamin D.

    The surgical correction of bile duct obstruction.

correlate *v.* to show a causal relationship

    The presence of ankylosing spondylitis correlates strongly with the B27 antigen.

correlation *n.* a causal relationship between two things

    A close, good ⟷ poor, high ⟷ low, strong ⟷ weak, good, positive ⟷ negative; significant correlation.

correspondingly *adv.* in agreement, in proportion

    As external pressure increases, the pressure of gas in the lungs increases correspondingly.

co-secrete *vt.* to secrete two substances at the same time

    These cancer cells co-secrete prolactin and growth hormone.

cosmetic *adj.* relating to appearance or correction of unsightly defects

    Cosmetic surgery.

cosmetically *adv.* from the cosmetic point of view

    Cosmetically unacceptable tumours.

counsel *vt.* to give advice and support

    She was counselled early in pregnancy about the value of a nutritious diet.

counselling (BE), **counseling** (AE) *n.* advice and support

    These women had received adequate counselling before mastectomy.

count *n.* the act or result of calculation

    To /do/make/ a bacterial count on a specimen, a complete blood count on a patient.

counteract *vt.* to act against

    The effect of a drug may be counteracted by a specific antagonist.

counterproductive *adj.* contrary to what is desired

    The treatment had a counterproductive effect.

couple *vt.* to link

    Ethanol oxidation is coupled with the reduction of oxaloacetic acid to malate.

course *n.*

    1. progression of a disease

    A disease may follow, have, pursue, run, an asymptomatic,

benign, fatal, fulminant, fulminating, prolonged, relentlessly progressive, self-limited (= self-limiting), unremitting course.

A treatment modifies, shortens the course of a disease.

The natural /course/history/ of a gastric ulcer.

This sign occurs late in the course of the disease.

2. a course of a drug or other treatment

All patients completed the course.

They received variable courses of prednisone treatment.

A protracted hospital course.

Short-course chemotherapy.

3. a mode of action

The best course was to reassure the patient.

co-worker, coworker *n.* a fellow research worker

Brown and (his) co-workers.

Compare: *et al.*

crave *vt.* to desire intensely

Patients taking lorazepam tended to crave (for) their next tablet.

craving *n.* an intense desire

Gastrointestinal bleeding causes a craving to chew ice.

To /have a craving for/crave (for)/ something.

crippling *adj.* causing serious disablement

Alcoholism is a crippling disorder.

crisis *n.* a turning point in the course of a disease with subsequent worsening or improvement in the patient's condition

An acute rejection crisis.

To /induce/trigger/ a crisis.

criterion *n.* (pl. criteria); a standard of evaluation

To adopt certain criteria for diagnosis.

To /fulfil/meet/satisfy/ criteria.

The diagnosis was made on clinical and radiological criteria.

Compare: arbiter, grounds, guide

critical *adj.*

1. involving a crisis

Critical condition.

2. decisive

This mechanism is critical to the action of the digitalis glycosides.

cross *vi.*

1. to move across

Iodine crosses the placental barrier.

Compare: pass

2. to move (a patient) to a parallel treatment group

Patients received two tablets of either placebo or the drug daily for four weeks and were then crossed (over) to the alternative preparation for a further four weeks.

cross-over *adj.*

1. changing of places

The mean blood pressure in women is lower than in men in younger adult life and higher in late middle life and beyond, the cross-over occurring typically at ages 40 to 54.

2. of a study in which patients are used as their own controls

The trial was of a cross-over /design/type. Each patient was given one drug for four weeks and then another for a further four weeks. The individual sequence was determined on a random basis.

A cross-over comparison.

cross-sectional *adj.* of a study involving a representative sample investigating at a specific point of time

In cross-sectional nutritional studies, different age groups are studied at the same time, whereas in longitudinal studies, the same persons are studied at the same time (during follow-up).

crucial *adj.* of decisive importance

Clearing the airways is crucial for the treatment of respiratory failure.

Compare: critical

crude *adj.* producing approximate results

A crude assay.

Crude estimated years of survival.

culminate *vi.* to reach its highest point

The anaphylactic reaction culminated in cardiac arrest.

culture *n.*

1. The reproduction of microorganisms or living tissue in prepared media capable of sustaining life and growth

To discharge, send, take material or a swab for culture.

2. the result of culturing, a growth

To establish cell cultures from skin specimens.

To obtain, take cultures for (the detection of) viral disease.

Bacterial cultures of blood were negative in these patients = They had negative cultures for the bacteria.

Cultures of these specimens yielded tubercle bacilli.

culture *vt.* to grow

The pathogen was cultured from asymptomatic carriers, needle aspirations, the blood.

Compare: isolate, recover

cumbersome *adj.* laborious

This assay is too cumbersome for large-scale studies.

Compare: laborious

curable *adj.* that can be cured
A curable disease; surgically curable tumours.
Opposite: incurable
curability *n.* the capacity for being cured
The curability of a disease.
curative *adj.* effecting a cure
A curative operation.
This treatment may be helpful but it is curative only in mild cases.
cure *n.*
1. a return to health, the successful treatment of a disease
To /achieve/bring about/effect/ a cure by treatment.
The treatment /brought about a cure/was curative/.
To seek cure for a disease.
Long-term cure was /achieved/attained/obtained/ by this treatment.
The cure rate of a treatment.
2. an effective drug or a treatment.
There is no cure for this disease.
3. a course or period of treatment
She took a cure for drug dependence.
cure *vt.* to bring or return to health
He was cured by antibiotic treatment.
He was cured of his leukaemia.
current *adj.*
1. prevailing, commonly accepted
The /current consensus/the contemporary view/ is that cardiac pacing is necessary in these patients.
According to current understanding.
2. available at present
Current evidence supports this concept.
3. in progress
These antibody titres indicate a /current/ongoing (AE)/ infection.
currently *adv.* at present
The drug is /currently/now/ under investigation for the treatment of meningitis.
cytopathic *adj.* causing pathological changes in a cell
The HIV virus is cytopathic to its target T4 cell.

D

damage *n.* harm

Damage from prolonged high blood pressure.

Heavy, severe ⟷ slight damage due to disease.

Radiation damage.

To /cause/do/ damage to a nerve = to damage a nerve.

Note: **damage** is singular in ME. **damages** means monetary compensation imposed by law for causing damage.

Compare: destruction, harm

damage *vt.* to cause harm

His bronchi had been damaged by bronchitis.

dangerous *adj.* causing risk

The dangerous complications of pregnancy.

data *n.* facts, information

Data/accumulated/derived/obtained/ from animal models.

Data /in/on/ patients with hypertension.

Data on the genetic transmission of this disease are scanty, meagre ⟷ abundant.

To /collect/elicit/gain/ data by interviewing a patient.

Originally a Latin plural word, **data** is now often considered singular. It is sometimes replaceable by **facts**, **results** or **values**.

Compare: finding, observation, result, value

date *n.* the present moment

This is the largest study of melanomas to be published /to date/ so far/.

Up-to-date/modern/ laboratory equipment.

dates *n.* the calculated gestation of a fetus

A small-for-dates baby.

death *n.*

1. the end of life

The disease is invariably fatal, with death usually resulting from hepatic failure.

Death from asthma = death due to asthma.

Death in these children usually is a result of vasculitis.

Death is imminent in patients with airway obstruction.

Death occurred after two months.

To ascertain the cause of death.

The death rate in these patients = the mortality rate.

2. an instance of this

Deaths associated with an infection.

Deaths attributable to an infection.

debatable *adj*. open to question

The efficacy of this treatment is debatable.

Compare: disputable

debate *n*. dispute

The exact mechanism of this effect remains a /source/subject/ of debate.

Compare: controversy, disagreement, dispute

debate *vi. vt*. to argue about

To debate (/on/about/) something with somebody.

The exact cause of the disease is still debated.

debilitated *adj*. weakened

Debilitated patients.

debilitating *adj*. weakening

Prolonged fever is debilitating.

v. debilitate

decelerate *vi. vt*. to (cause to) reduce speed

Their growth rate had decelerated.

A /decelerating/slowing/ growth rate.

Opposites: accelerate, speed

Compare: retard

deceleration *n*. reduction of speed

They showed a progressive deceleration of growth rate.

Opposite: acceleration

Compare: retardation

declare *vt*. to show

His diabetes had /declared/simply: shown/ itself clinically.

Compare: manifest, show

decline *n*. decrease, deterioration

A /decline/decrease/ in the number of patients.

The mental /decline/deterioration/ of Huntington's chorea.

decline *vi. vt*.

1. *vi*. to become smaller (in amount)

The incidence of these side-effects declined progressively.

Compare: decrease

2. *vi*. to become worse

Appetite, health may decline.

Compare: deteriorate

3. *vt*. to refuse

One patient declined participation in the study, further interview.

Compare: refuse

decompensation *n*. inability to maintain adequate function

Hepatic decompensation may lead to hepatic coma.

Compare: failure, insufficiency

decrease *n.* diminution

    1. the process of diminution

    A decrease in length.

    To be on the decrease = to be decreasing.

    2. the amount of diminution

    A decrease of 20 ml, 20%.

decrease *vi. vt.* to (cause to) become smaller, by a definite or non-definite amount

    To decrease by a unit of measure (by 20 ml, 20%).

    To decrease from something to something (from 500 ml to 300 ml).

    To decrease in length.

    to be decreased = often simply: to be lower, to be less

    Note: **decrease** like many other verbs of change is often used in the passive:

    The relative volume of the mitochondria was decreased.

    Compare: decline, drop, fall, wane; lower, reduce

decrement *n.* a small decrease

    Small decrements of dosage.

    Opposite: increment

deep *adj.* located far from the surface

    Deep tissues, veins.

deeply *adv.* far down from the surface

    The ulcer had penetrated deeply.

deep-seated *adj.* deep

    Deep-seated tumours.

default *vi.* to fail to participate or comply

    He defaulted on follow-up.

    He defaulted the trial for social reasons.

    The default rate for the group was high.

    n. default, defaulter

defect *n.* an imperfection or lack; failure

    To have a defect in a function, in an organ.

    To correct a defect.

    A genetic defect; a methodological defect.

defective *adj.* showing a defect

    Defective immunity.

defence (BE), **defense** (AE) *n.* resistance (against infection)

    IgG provides the body's main serological defences against bacteria.

deficiency *n.* a defect

    A deficiency disease is any specific pathological state, with characteristic clinical signs, that is due to an insufficient intake of energy or essential nutrients (WHO 1).

Dietary deficiency (⟵⟶ excess) of folic acid.

Hormonal deficiency.

The study had some methodological deficiencies.

Compare: defect, deficit

deficient *adj.* having none or not enough of; lacking in

Folic acid was deficient in both patients = Both patients were deficient in folic acid.

Studies deficient in methodology.

Thiamine-deficient patients = patients deficient in thiamine.

deficit *n.* a defect

Alzheimer's disease is principally manifested by memory deficits.

A deficit /in/of/ folic acid.

A neurological deficit.

Compare: deficiency

definable *adj.* that can be defined

A clinically definable group of epilepsies.

define *vt.*

1. to state the meaning of

We tried to define vascular resistance in terms of cardiac dynamics.

2. to determine the nature or limits of

The maternal groups were defined by planned place of delivery.

definition *n.*

1. a statement of the meaning of a word

The definition of coma.

2. determination of the nature or limits of

A more precise definition of the heart lesion was needed.

degrade *vt.* to reduce the complexity of a chemical compound

These fragments are degraded into much smaller peptides.

degree *n.* the extent, measure, grade or scope of an effect (such as disease)

Patients with different degrees of congestive heart failure.

His anaemia was moderate in degree = briefly: His anaemia was moderate.

delayed-acting *adj.* acting slowly

Delayed-acting tablets.

delete *vt.* to remove

Adriamycin was deleted from the treatment to avoid cardiac toxicity.

n. deletion

deleterious *adj.* harmful

Deleterious/usually: harmful/ histological changes in the liver.

Compare: detrimental, harmful, injurious

deletion *n.* the act of deleting

Deletion of a drug from the treatment.

delineate *vt.* to describe (accurately)

We tried to delineate the morphological variations of chronic lymphocytic anaemia.

n. delineation

deliver *vt.*

1. to supply

To deliver oxygen to an organ.

2. to give birth to a child

She delivered a healthy child vaginally.

delivery *n.*

1. supply

The delivery of a drug to its site of action.

The delivery of oxygen to tissues.

Compare: supply

2. giving birth to a child

Assisted delivery.

demand *n.* requirement

The oxygen demand of a tissue.

Compare: requirement

demand *vt.* to need urgently

Severe interstitial cystitis may demand cystectomy.

Compare: require

demarcate *vt.* to mark the limits of

A sharply demarcated inflammation.

n. demarcation

Compare: circumscribe, define, delineate

demonstrable *adj.* that can be demonstrated

The tumour was demonstrable on bronchoscopic examination.

demonstrate *vt.*

1. to show the existence of

Parasites were demonstrated in the blood.

Compare: find, show

2. to develop, have, show signs and symptoms

The patient demonstrated allergy to drugs.

Compare: show

demonstration *n.* the act, process or result of demonstrating

The diagnosis of this disease /depends/rests/ on the demonstration of parasites in skin snips or nodules.

de novo *adv.* from the beginning, with no precedent

Lymphomas arising de novo ⟷ lymphomas presenting as metastases.

Compare: primary

denial *n.* declaration of the untruthfulness of a proposition

The denial of drinking is often based on guilt or fear.

deny *vt.* to declare untrue

She denied alcohol abuse.

She denied having taken the drug.

Opposites: admit, affirm

depend *vi.* to rely on, require

The commonest tests for glycosuria depend on copper reduction.

The heart depends on coronary blood flow for sustained normal function.

dependence *n.* the condition of being dependent

Alcohol, drug dependence.

A dependence-producing drug.

Dependence on nicotine.

Compare: drug dependence

dependent *adj.* depending

These biochemical changes may be age- and sex-dependent.

Vitamin-D-dependent rickets.

Dependent on ⟷ independent of.

To be dependent on = often simply: to depend on.

depict *vt.* to represent (by a picture, an image), describe

Computed tomography scanning may depict the thoracic contents.

deplete *vt.* to empty partially or totally

He was /depleted of fluid/dehydrated.

depletion *n.* the process or result of depleting

Electrolyte depletion.

The depletion of the body's iron stores.

deposit *n.* an accumulation of

The liver contained secondary deposits of cancer.

deposit *vi. vt.* to accumulate

Porphyrins had deposited in the skin.

depress *vt.*

1. to lower, weaken

Protein binding is depressed in uraemia.

Sedatives may depress respiration.

Depressed blood phosphate concentrations, myocardial blood flow.

2. to sadden, discourage

The death of a near relative had depressed him.

depression *n.*

1. the abnormal lowering of a value

Depressions in aspartate transaminase values.

2. reduction in activity

Bone marrow depression.

3. a psychotic disorder marked by 'anhedonia, and features such as sad, mournful look, tears, gloomy tone of voice, deep sighing, and choking of voice on depressing topic' (WHO 2)

Distinguishing dementia from depression may be difficult.

depressive *adj.* pertaining to depression

Depressive delusions, neurosis.

The depressive action of high serum calcium levels on the autonomic nervous system.

deprived of *adj.* lacking in

An infant deprived of fluid may lose 4% of its body weight per day.

Compare: depleted of

deputize, deputise *vi.* to act on behalf of other staff

A medical emergency deputizing service operated outside normal surgery hours.

Compare: call, duty

derange *vt.* to disturb (especially of mental processes)

The higher mental processes may be deranged diffusely or focally.

derangement *n.* abnormality

Metabolic derangement (e.g. renal failure, diabetes).

Compare: abnormality, disturbance

derivative *n.* a compound derived from a structurally related compound

A synthetic derivative of vitamin A.

derive *vi. vt.*

1. *vi. vt.* to (cause to) be drawn from

Phytohaemagglutinin is derived from bean plants.

Serum IgA may derive from secretory IgA.

A derived drug (= a derivative) $\longleftrightarrow$ a parent drug.

2. *vt.* to obtain

To derive data from studies.

They derived an excellent result from this treatment.

Compare: obtain

describe *vt.* to give an account of

Chronic recurrent multifocal osteomyelitis was first described in 1972.

n. description

descriptive *adj.* serving to describe

The term is descriptive of the pathophysiology of this disease.

design *n.* a study plan

The study /followed/had/ an open, randomized, balanced, cross-over design.

design *vt.* to plan (a study)
A retrospective study was designed.

designate *vt.* to categorize, diagnose
These cases were designated as periarteritis nodosa.
Compare: categorize, classify, diagnose, label

desirable *adj.* having beneficial properties
The drug may be desirable in these cases.
Opposite: undesirable
Compare: beneficial

destroy *vt.* to make useless, put an end to
This enzyme may destroy various penicillins.

destruction *n.* the act or result of destroying
A virus can cause destruction in a cell in many ways.
Irreversible renal destruction.
Compare: damage

detachment *n.* the separation of a small unit from a larger body
The detachment of ciliated epithelium occurs in asthma.
v. detach

detect *vt.* to find (as a result of looking)
The tumour was detected /by/on/ colonoscopy.
To detect occult blood in the urine.
n. detection
Compare: disclose, find, reveal

detectable *adj.* that can be detected
The lesion was detectable by ultrasound.

deteriorate *vi. vt.* to (cause to) become worse
His health, his condition, deteriorated progressively.
n. deterioration
Compare: aggravate, decline, exacerbate, worsen

determination *n.* the process or result of determining a physical quantity
Serum glucose /determinations are made/is determined/ on a specimen from a fasting patient.
Compare: assay, assessment, estimation, evaluation, measurement

determine *vt.* to find out a value or a property by a series of observations (usually by means of laboratory tests)
ABO blood groups were determined from blood samples.
Compare: assay, assess, measure

detriment *n.* harm, damage
Alcohol is /a detriment/detrimental/ to health.
The detriments of a treatment.

detrimental *adj.* very harmful

The treatment had a detrimental effect.

Neurologically detrimental haemorrhages.

Opposite: beneficial

develop *vi. vt.*

1. *vi. vt.* to (cause to) grow or increase to a later or more advanced stage

Polyps may develop into cancer.

To develop from one cell into an organism.

2. *vi. vt.* to acquire or begin to occur (abruptly or gradually)

Drug addicts may develop small septic emboli from endocarditis. = Small septic emboli may develop in drug addicts . . .

n. development

3. *vt.* to elaborate

To develop a method.

developer *n.* one who develops (a disease)

Premature or early developers of coronary heart disease.

development *n.*

1. a later stage

Bacteraemia is a dangerous development in any infection.

2. gradual acquisition

The development of pustules.

3. elaboration

The development of kidney transplantation in man.

deviation *n.* divergence

A deviation from linearity.

devoid *adj.* devoid of = lacking in

The technique is not /devoid of/simply: without/ risk.

diagnose *vt.* to determine, identify, or distinguish the nature of a disease

He was diagnosed as having cystic fibrosis.

The case was correctly, erroneously/incorrectly/mistakenly/wrongly/; presumptively, provisionally, tentatively diagnosed as cystic fibrosis.

He was diagnosed from the history and clinical examination.

He was diagnosed on clinical grounds.

To diagnose by /exclusion/elimination/.

adj. diagnosable

diagnosis *n.* the identification of a disease in a patient

The diagnosis /was based/rested/ on arteriography, on the demonstration of pericardial calcification.

The diagnosis was /confirmed/substantiated/ by laboratory tests.

The diagnosis was entertained in two patients.

The diagnosis was /established/made/ at laparotomy, /on/by/ biopsy, by examining samples.

The diagnosis was indicated by the presence of certain signs.

The diagnosis was inferred, made from findings.

The diagnosis was made from a history of an animal bite, from amniotic fluid, by history and examination, on histological grounds.

The diagnosis was /missed/overlooked/ because of administrative errors.

The diagnosis was refuted, excluded.

He /was given/received/ a diagnosis of prostatic cancer.

It was difficult to /arrive at/reach/ a correct diagnosis.

A diagnosis can be certain, correct, definitive, doubtful, false, firm, erroneous, incorrect, obvious, presumptive, provisional or tentative.

The diagnosis was evident from the history.

ECG evidence in this infant favoured a diagnosis of fibroelastosis.

Differential diagnosis = the differentiation of one disease from another in diagnosis.

diagnostic *adj.*

1. relating to diagnosis

Diagnostic accuracy, errors, procedures, /results/yield/.

This test is a valuable diagnostic tool.

To draw diagnostic conclusions from the history.

2. evidence for making a diagnosis

Koplik's spots are diagnostic of measles.

The CF test is diagnostic at a titre of about 1:64.

Compare: compatible, pathognomonic

diagnostically *adv.* from the diagnostic point of view

A diagnostically high plasma insulin concentration.

diagrammatically *adv.* by means of diagram(s)

The results of the study were presented diagrammatically.

n. diagram

diary *n.* a daily record of symptoms, etc.

Patients recorded subjective progress by completing a diary giving details of symptoms.

dictate *vt.* to determine

The choice of liver biopsy technique is dictated by the coagulation state of the patient.

dictum *n.* a formal saying

It is better to prevent disease than to cure it is a commonsense medical dictum.

die *vi.* to cease biological activity

To die from asthma, starvation.

To die of a disease.

Patients dying in congestive heart failure.

Patients dying with disseminated malignant disease, with shock.

Euphemisms to be avoided: expire, pass away, succumb

diet *n.* the total solid and liquid foods consumed by an individual or a population group, either on an average basis or during a specified period. A special schedule for eating and drinking, usually prescribed by a physician or a dietician (WHO 1).

Kinds of diet: balanced, bland, easily digestible, diabetic, elimination, experimental, high ⟷ low calorie, high- ⟷ low-fibre, high- ⟷ low-residue, (routine) hospital, lactose-free, liquid, low-fat, low-salt, prescribed, proper, protein-free, recommended, restricted, strict ⟷ relaxed or test diet.

A diet based on milk, a diet /high/rich/ in purines.

To /adhere to/follow/ the prescribed diet.

To exclude a food from the diet.

To maintain a patient on a diet, to put a patient on a diet.

dietary *adj.*

1. relating to an ordinary diet

Dietary requirements of vitamins, dietary sources of carbo-hydrates.

2. relating to a prescribed diet

A dietary /plan/programme/ directed toward control of serum cholesterol concentrations.

Dietary allowances, compliance, recommendations.

To impose dietary restrictions.

differ from *vi.* to be unlike in nature, quality, degree

They did not differ from the other donors in age or sex.

difference *n.* the state or quality of being dissimilar; an instance of this

A difference of form, nature, quality, degree, etc. between two things.

A great ⟷ slight; striking difference.

Significant differences were found in favour of active treatment.

different *adj.* partly or completely unlike

Different from (BE, and formal AE).

This substance acts in a different way from nitrates.

differential *adj.* distinguishing

Differential diagnosis between two diseases by a method means the determination of which one of two or more similar diseases a person suffers from.

differentiate *vt.* to mark or show a difference between
To differentiate one disease from another by a method.
differentiation *n.* the act or process of differentiating
Differentiation between A and B by findings, by a method.
Differentiation of one disease from another.
diffuse *adj.* not definitely limited or localized; diffused
Diffuse abdominal tenderness.
diffuse *vi. vt.* to spread; to move down a concentration gradient
Most antibacterial agents do not diffuse from plasma into prostatic fluid.
n. diffusion
diffusible *adj.* that can be diffused
Carbon dioxide is highly diffusible.
dilate *vi. vt.*
1. to become wider
The blood vessels dilated in response to nitroglycerine.
Dilated pupils.
2. to make wider
To dilate an obstructed blood vessel.
dilatation (mainly BE), **dilation** (mainly AE) *n.* dilating or being dilated
Dilatation of blood vessels, of the pupils.
Dilatation/dilation/ of the uterine cervix.
dilemma *n.* a difficult problem of choice between two alternatives
This disease often poses a diagnostic dilemma.
Compare: problem
dilute *vi. vt.* to (cause to) become less concentrated
The samples were diluted /one in eight/eightfold/.
dilution *n.* a diluted solution
The antiseptic was applied in a 1:1000 dilution.
diminish *vi. vt.* to (cause to) become smaller in number or size
The body magnesium stores were diminished.
Compare: abate, decline, decrease, deplete
diminution *n.* reduction, decrease
A diminution /in/of/ operative mortality.
Compare: abatement, decline, decrease, depletion
direct *adj.* with nothing between
A direct symptom = a symptom directly due to the disease.
direct *vt.* to regulate an activity, a course towards a goal
The action of antibodies is directed against antigen.
disability *n.* any restriction or lack (resulting from an impairment) of ability to perform in the manner or within the range considered normal for a human being (WHO 2)
Disability in colour recognition, in understanding speech.

Personal safety disability includes leaving fires on (WHO 2).
Compare: handicap, impairment

disablement *n*. the state of a person with a disability; disability

disabling *adj*. causing disablement

A /disabling/incapacitating/ disease.

Disabling pain.

disadvantage *n*. an unfavourable, inferior condition or position

There are well-documented disadvantages /in/to/ the use of this treatment.

disagree *vi*. to lack agreement

Many authorities disagree on the importance of this symptom.

Other verbs expressing disagreement between research workers or their results: conflict, contradict, debate, disagree, diverge, vary

disagreement *n*. absence of agreement

Our findings are in disagreement with those of previous studies.

Other nouns expressing disagreement: conflict, contradiction, controversy, debate, discord, discrepancy, disparity, dispute divergence, variance

Adjectives expressing disagreement between results or workers: controversial, debatable, discordant, discrepant, disputable, divergent, variable

disappointing *adj*. failing to meet expectations

Intravenous urograms in young infants are often disappointing and sometimes dangerous.

Opposites: encouraging

Compare: discouraging, frustrating

discard *vt*. to dispose of

The uppermost layer of cells was discarded.

discharge *n*.

1. the act of discharging a liquid

Slight ⟷ copious discharge of pus from a wound.

2. the conclusion of a period of inpatient care in a hospital

At/on/ discharge, patients were advised to limit their animal fat intake.

Premature discharge from hospital.

Opposite: admission, hospitalization

discharge *vt*.

1. to pour or let out liquid

The wound discharged pus.

2. to allow to leave (hospital)

He was discharged on orally administered iron.

He was discharged to attend as an outpatient.

disclose *vt.* to reveal, show

A chest roentgenogram /disclosed/simply: showed/ pneumonia.

Compare: divulge, reveal, show

disclosure *n.* the act or result of disclosing

The patient's frank disclosure of his real level of alcohol consumption.

discomfort *n.* mental or physical uneasiness, (mild) pain

Gastrointestinal discomfort.

Headache is one of man's most frequent discomforts.

He was in considerable /discomfort/pain/.

Compare: distress

discontinue *vi. vt.* to stop

The drug was discontinued in five patients on account of adverse effects.

Compare: cease, withhold

discordant *adj.* lacking agreement

The results of the two studies were discordant.

Compare: conflicting, contradictory, divergent

discount *vt.* to rule out

We discounted (the possibility of) meningitis as the cause of the lesion.

discourage *vt.* to try to prevent an action by advice

Indiscriminate use of antibiotics should be discouraged.

She was discouraged from pushing until the cervix was fully dilated.

Opposites: advocate, encourage

discouraging *adj.* frustrating

Discouraging results.

discover *vt.* to find something existing but not known before

Carcinoma of the cervix is discovered by examination.

Koch discovered the phenomenon of delayed hypersensitivity to tuberculosis

To discover a new drug.

n. discovery

Compare: detect, find

discrepancy *n.* lack of agreement

A striking discrepancy between our results and those of others.

Compare: disagreement

discrepant *adj.* conflicting

Discrepant reports regarding the efficacy of this treatment.

discrete *adj.* distinct

A discrete space-occupying lesion.

Compare: discreet = careful, tactful

discriminant *n.* a distinguishing factor
This clinical feature is a useful discriminant in diagnosis.
Compare: criterion

discriminate *vt.* to distinguish
The test discriminates reliably between these two diseases.
Compare: differentiate, distinguish, separate

discuss *vt.* to debate, to treat a subject in speech or writing
To discuss a theme.

discussion *n.* the examination or consideration of a matter
The book contained a discussion of ethical issues.
The patient /under discussion/in question.

disease *n.* a pathological change identified after diagnosis
Pathology refers to the study of disease, particularly the changes causing or caused by disease. A disease causes illness in an individual.
To suffer from a disease.
Compare: ailment, complaint, disorder, illness, sickness

diseased *adj.* affected by disease, involved by disease
A diseased subject.
The diseased area was dissected.

disequilibrium *n.* see p. 115 under imbalance.

disintegration *n.* breaking into constituent elements
Timed-disintegration capsules.
v. disintegrate

disorder *n.* a form of malfunctioning
Disorders of ovarian function = ovarian dysfunction.
Disorders of the carbohydrate metabolism.
Learning /disorders/handicaps/ at school age.

disordered *adj.* disturbed
Disordered blood flow to the nodules contributes to portal hypertension.

disorientation *n.* mental confusion
The patient was suffering from disorientation in time and place.
adj. disoriented

disparity *n.* discrepancy
Disparity between physical and chest x-ray findings.
Compare: disagreement, discrepancy

display *vt.* to show, have
The rats /displayed/had/ high drug plasma concentrations.
Compare: show

disposable *adj.* intended to be used only once and then thrown away
Disposable syringes.

disposal *n.* elimination

Plasma magnesium affected the disposal of glucose loads from the blood.

dispose of *vi.* to remove, eliminate

Urinary excretion will dispose of excess urea.

disproportionate *adj.* out of proportion

The enlargement of the left atrium was disproportionate to that of the left ventricle.

disproportionately *adv.* out of proportion

A disproportionately enlarged left atrium.

disprove *vt.* to prove (something) to be incorrect

Tomography disproved the presence of a tumour.

dispute *n.* a debate, disagreement

The matter is /in/under/ dispute.

In dispute with = in disagreement with; without dispute = undoubtedly

adj. disputable

disregard *vt.* to exclude in diagnosis

To disregard a diagnostic possibility.

Compare: discount, eliminate, exclude, rule out

disrupt *vt.*

1. to cause to break down

These lesions disrupt neural connections.

Vinblastine disrupts the morphology of the parathyroid gland.

Compare: destroy

2. to throw into disorder

Hospital patients have a disrupted lifestyle.

n. disruption

disruptive *adj.* causing disruption

The treatment /was disruptive of/plainly: disrupted/ the patient's life.

dissect *vt.*

1. to cut apart

A strip of endothelium was dissected from the uterine cervix.

2. separate and expose, especially cadaveric tissues for ana-tomical studies

n. Dissection.

disseminate *vi.* to spread over a wide area

The malignant cells had disseminated throughout the body.

adj. disseminated, diffuse ⟷ localized

dissimilar *adj.* not similar

The lesions of sarcoidosis are dissimilar to the mass in this patient.

dissolve *vi. vt.* to (cause to) pass into solution

The modern formulations of digoxin dissolve rapidly.

The powder was dissolved in water.
Compare: disintegrate
n. dissolution

dissuade *vt.* to advise against
Doctors should try to dissuade pregnant women from smoking.
Compare: discourage
n. dissuasion

distal *adj.* farther away from the point of reference
Arterial pressure was measured both proximal and distal to the obstruction.
Opposite: proximal

distend *vt.* to expand
The bowel was distended with gas.

distension, distention *n.* the act or result of expanding
Abdominal distension.

distinction *n.* a difference
To /draw/make/ a distinction between two diseases on the basis of clinical findings.

distinguish *vt.* to make or recognize differences
This assay should distinguish between HSV-1 and HSV-2 infections.
These enzymes can be distinguished by their kinetic properties.
The productive cough of chronic bronchitis should be distinguished from chronic airway obstruction.
The distinguishing features of a disease.
adj. distinguishable
Compare: differentiate, separate

distort *vt.*
1. to cause false results
This agent distorts thyroid function tests.
2. to pull or twist out of the natural, usual, or original shape
The lesion had /distorted/disrupted/ the cell architecture of the liver.

distortion *n.* alteration by distorting
The distortion of lung architecture.

distress *n.*
1. physical pain, strain
He was in acute distress on admission.
Respiratory distress.
Compare: discomfort
2. emotional anguish, mental pain
To /alleviate/ease/mitigate/ emotional distress.

Compare: discomfort
3. a state of danger
Fetal distress.

distribute *vt*. to give out parts of a whole
To distribute along a line, over an area, throughout a volume, among individuals, or in a tissue.

distribution *n*. the result of distributing
Rotaviruses have a world-wide distribution.
Three joints were affected by arthritis in an uneven distribution.

disturbance *n*. the state or an instance of being disturbed physically or mentally
Disturbance of blood flow, mental disturbance.
Severe constitutional disturbances occurred at this high temperature.
Compare: derangement

disturbed *adj*.
1. suffering from a change in its natural or usual condition
Disturbed blood flow.
2. showing symptoms of emotional illness
Mentally disturbed patients.

disturbing *adj*. (unexpected and) upsetting
This study gave disturbing results.

diurnal *adj*. occurring during one day
Diurnal variations.
Compare: circadian

divergent *adj*. different
Divergent opinions.
Compare: different

divide *vi*. *vt*. to separate or be separated
To divide into several different quantities or categories.
To subdivide = to divide further.
n. division of something into parts

divulge *vt*. to disclose confidential or personal matters
A patient divulges information at interview.
Compare: disclose, reveal

do *vi*. *vt*.
1. *vt*. to carry out
To do an assay, an autopsy, a biopsy, a blood count, damage, a determination, an examination, harm, an operation, a procedure, research, sampling, staining, a study, surgery, a test, a trial.
Quantitative x-ray studies were done on these vertebrae.
Compare: carry out, conduct, make

2. *vi.* to fare

Postoperatively the patient did poorly ⟷ well, satisfactorily.

document *vt.*

1. to support with evidence from investigations

Fluoroscopically documented paralysis of the diaphragm.

The use of this treatment in pneumonia is /widely/well/ ⟷ poorly/ documented.

2. to record

It is essential at the time of diagnosis to document completely the extent of Hodgkin's disease.

documentation *n.* evidence in the form of documented investigations

Convincing laboratory documentation was lacking.

domiciliary *adj.* taking place in the patient's home

Domiciliary births = births at home = home births.

Domiciliary care ⟷ hospital or institutional care.

donor *n.* a person who donates tissue for use in the treatment of another

A histocompatible donor.

A living ⟷ cadaveric donor.

A living related donor.

Opposites: recipient; rarely: donee

dormant *adj.* inactive, quiescent; subclinical

dosage *n.* the amount of medicine given during a given period of time; BE usage: the giving, regulation or gradation of doses, seldom the amount taken at one time (=dose).

The drug was administered at a dosage of 1 mg twice a day.

They were controlled on a low dosage.

The high-dosage group.

To individualize dosage.

To increase ⟷ decrease, reduce dosage; dosage reduction.

dosage adjustment *n.* the adjustment of dosage

His ataxia was reversible by proper dosage adjustment.

dosage schedule *n.* dosage plan; dosage

One dose in the morning; a second dose administered 6 hours later. This dosage and dosage schedule can be maintained or even reduced.

Note: dosage scheme (frequently AE)

dose *n.* primary meaning: the amount of drug taken at one time

The drug is given as a single dose preferably in the morning.

Drowsiness occurred /at/with/ a dose of 300 mg.

The drug was injected at doses exceeding several times the usual therapeutic dose of 20–40 mg.

The drug was given/used in a dose depending on the patient's weight.

The optimum dose was 80–160 mg/day in divided doses.

They were treated adequately with a lower dose.

To /decrease/reduce/taper/ ⟷ increase/ a dose by 20% decrements ⟷ increments

Individually determined single doses.

An initial dose = a starting dose.

A maintenance dose.

Patients on high-dose, middle-dose or low-dose therapy.

Compare: dosage

dose-dependent *adj.* dependent on the dose

A dose-dependent impairment of antibody production.

dose-related *adj.* related to the dose

This type of agranulocytosis may be dose-related to the administration of alkylating agents.

double-blind *adj.* of a clinical trial in which neither the observer nor the test subject knows the nature of the treatment

The trial was conducted in double-blind fashion.

The trial was double-blind with randomization of placebo and drug.

A double-blind ⟷ open trial.

Compare: single-blind trial

doubt *n.* uncertainty about a belief or opinion

Serious doubts have been /expressed/raised/ about the wisdom of this treatment policy.

drain *vi. vt.* to empty

A blood vessel or the blood in it drains into another blood vessel.

A rich supply of lymphatic vessels drains the liver.

drainage *n.* withdrawal of fluids

The drainage of a wound.

dramatic *adj.* striking

A dramatic improvement in the patient's condition.

Dramatic and *striking* are usually used about an increase or improvement, while *drastic* is used about a decrease or deterioration.

dramatically *adv.* in a dramatic way

The patient responded dramatically to treatment.

draw *vt.* to extract

Blood was drawn for assessments of the hormone.

Compare: collect

dreaded *adj.* greatly feared

Retinopathy is a dreaded complication of diabetes.

dress *vt.* to apply protective or therapeutic bandage, ointment, etc.
To dress a wound with gauze.
n. dressing

drip *n.* drop by drop infusion of a liquid or the necessary apparatus
The drug was given by continuous intragastric drip.
He was maintained on a drip for 24 hours.

drop-out *n.*
1. withdrawal (during a trial or investigation)
The drop-out rate on placebo was low.
Compare: default, non-compliance
2. a subject who defaults a trial = a defaulter

drop out *vi.* to default during a trial
Two patients treated with placebo dropped out within four weeks.

drug *n.*
1. any substance administered to man for the prophylaxis, diagnosis or therapy of disease or for the modification of physiological function (WHO 1).
He had one month's treatment on this drug.
A prescription drug: a pharmaceutical speciality which can be obtained by the public on prescription only (WHO 1).
An over-the-counter drug: a pharmaceutical speciality which can be obtained by the public without prescription (WHO 1).
A proprietary drug: a drug marketed under a trademark (WHO 1).
A non-proprietary drug/a generic drug/: a drug marketed otherwise than under a trademark (i.e. under its scientific name) (WHO 1).
2. a substance used for non-medical purposes and capable of producing drug dependence or other undesirable effects (WHO 1)
He is dependent on hallucinogenic drugs.

drug abuse *n.* the consumption of a drug apart from medical need or in unnecessary quantities (WHO 1)

drug-related *adj.* involving a drug
Drug-related deaths, toxicities.

drug-resistant *adj.* resistant to the action of drugs
A drug-resistant microorganism.

due to *adj.* ascribable to
Disease A is due to factor B = Factor B is responsible for disease A.
due to the fact that = shorter: because

dull *vt.* to make less intense or less keen
An analgesic agent dulls pain.

Overuse of this drug may dull alertness.

duration *n.* the length of time during which something exists or continues

Disease duration.

The duration of drug action, survival after transplantation.

The duration of treatment.

duty *n.* a service allocated

To be on /duty/call/.

At night the duty consultant anaesthetist and duty consultant physician covered the intensive care unit.

dying *adj.* see: die, moribund

dysfunction *n.* impaired functioning

Dysfunction of the endothelium.

Left ventricular dysfunction.

Ovarian dysfunction, menstrual dysfunction.

dysfunctional *adj.* relating to dysfunction

Dysfunctional uterine bleeding.

E

early *adj.* occurring during the initial stages of
    Early detection of disease by screening.
    Early ⟷ late postoperative complications.
    Findings in early breast cancer.
    Compare: premature
educate *vt.* to teach
    Couples should be educated about their job as parents and
    taught about child development and children's needs.
    To educate a patient in home dialysis techniques
    Compare: instruct
education *n.* instruction
    Improved patient education about asthma is needed.
    The education of a patient in understanding his disease.
    The education of mothers for childbirth.
effect *n.* the result of an action
    The treatment /exerts/has/produces/provides/ an effect on
    lymphocytes.
    To sustain an effect.
    Peak analgesic effects developed at about 45 min.
    The effect of a drug wears off.
    The effect of this drug is related to its hypotensive property.
    Compare: action, efficacy, influence, potency; sequel, side-effect
effect *vt.* to bring about
    To effect a change.
    Compare: to affect something = to have an effect on something
effective *adj.* producing a desired effect
    The drug is effective /against/for/ seizures.
    The drug is effective in multiple myeloma.
    The procedure is effective in restoring T-cell immunity.
    The lowest effective dose.
    Compare: efficacious, potent
effectiveness *n.* the ability to produce an effect
    To assess the effectiveness of a drug in a trial
    Compare: efficacy
efficacious *adj.* effective
    An efficacious drug or treatment.
    Compare: effective
efficacy *n.* the benefit or utility to the individual of the services,

treatment regimen, drug, preventive or control measure advocated or applied (WHO 1)

The efficacy of a drug /for/in/ maintenance therapy.

efficient *adj.* functioning effectively, competent

An efficient surgical team.

effusion *n.* the escape of fluid from anatomical vessels by rupture or exudation into a part or tissue

Chest radiography showed a large pleural effusion.

e.g. or **eg** *abbr.* for example

elaborate *vt.* to produce

Neurohumeral substances are elaborated in the anterior hypothalamus.

Compare: manufacture, produce, release

elaboration *n.* production

The elaboration of a hormone by a gland.

Compare: manufacture, production, release

elapse *vi.* (of time) to pass by

One hour had elapsed since the last injection.

The elapsed time.

elderly *adj.* past middle age

This procedure has a lower death rate notably in /the elderly/ elderly patients/.

elect *vt.* to choose voluntarily

She elected to have amniocentesis.

elective *adj.* decided on by the patient or physician

Elective abortion of a seriously malformed fetus.

Elective cessation of therapy.

Elective (caesarean) section.

Elective ⟷ emergency surgery.

elevate *vt.* to raise

Alkaline phosphatase activity was elevated.

The leucocyte count is often elevated in vasculitis.

n. elevation

Compare: increase, raise

elicit *vt.*

1. to draw out (information)

Chvostek's sign could not be elicited.

Side-effects of the drug were elicited with a questionnaire.

To elicit a family history from a patient at interview.

2. to produce

To elicit a reaction, a response.

Compare: obtain, produce, provoke

eligible *adj.* qualified for a treatment or a study

Ten patients were eligible for /enrolment/inclusion/ in the study.

Compare: candidate

Opposite: ineligible

eligibility *n*. qualifications

A subject's eligibility for a study.

Eligibility criteria.

eliminate *vt*. to remove

A drug is absorbed, metabolized and eliminated from the body.

To eliminate a disease from further consideration in diagnosis.

n. elimination

Compare: remove; rule out

elucidate *vt*. to clarify

The duration of these disturbances could not be elucidated by the present method.

The structure of insulin has been elucidated.

Compare: clarify, explain

n. elucidation

emanate *vi*. to proceed from a source

The epidemic /emanated from/could be traced back to/ a single index patient.

embarrass *vt*. to impair

This factor embarrasses cardiac function.

Compare: compromise, derange, disturb

embarrassment *n*. the impairment of a function

Circulatory, respiratory embarrassment.

Compare: compromise, failure, insufficiency

emerge *vi*. to appear, become known

New methods /emerge/are introduced.

emergency *n*.

1. an unexpected medical condition requiring immediate attention

Facial fractures are an emergency if there is any degree of airway obstruction.

Hypertensive emergency.

2. a patient requiring urgent treatment

He was admitted to hospital as an emergency.

emphasis *n*. special importance

To /lay/place/put/ emphasis on = to give emphasis to.

Compare: attach importance to, place stress on, stress something, underline

emphasize, emphasise *vt*.

1. to attach special importance to

Many reports emphasize the need to avoid shellfish.
The study emphasized the role of prophylaxis.
2. to intensify
Selegiline may emphasize the side-effects of levodopa.
Compare: accentuate, exaggerate

empirical, empiric *adj.* based on experience rather than theory
The amount of antitoxin given was based on an empirical decision.

employ *vt.* to use
To employ/simply: use/ a method.

empty *vi. vt.* to drain
The vena cava empties into the right atrium.
Compare: drain

enable *vt.* to make able or possible
To enable somebody to do something.
To enable something to be done = to allow something to be done.
Compare: allow, permit

en bloc *adv.* total or totally, in one piece
An en bloc excision.
To remove a tumour en bloc.

encompass *vt.* to discuss or include comprehensively
The author of the book tried to encompass immunology in 50 pages.

encounter *n.* a meeting
to /encounter/simply: have/ problems.
This disease /is encountered/occurs/ in the elderly.
A commonly encountered finding = simply: a common finding.
Compare: find

encourage *vt.* to advise
To encourage a patient to stop smoking.
n. encouragement ⟷ discouragement
Compare: advise

encouraging *adj.* promising
An encouraging finding.
Compare: gratifying, promising, rewarding
Opposites: disappointing, discouraging

encroach *vi.* to invade (insidiously)
The tumour had encroached on the sinuses.

encroachment *n.* insidious invasion
The encroachment of a tumour on bone marrow.

end-stage *adj.* terminal, terminating in death
End-stage renal disease.

engorge *vt.* to congest with fluid
>A segment of the right lobe was left without drainage and became engorged.
>*n.* engorgement

engulf *vt.* to destroy by swallowing up
>Particles of free silica are engulfed by alveolar macrophages.

enhance *vt.* to improve
>To enhance ⟷ suppress cell division.
>The drug may /enhance/potentiate/ the depressive effects of alcohol.
>*Compare*: augment, increase, improve, potentiate

enjoy *vt.* to have
>She /enjoyed/simply: had/ a normal pregnancy.
>She had /enjoyed/simply: had/ good health.

enlarge *vi. vt.* to make or become larger
>The swelling recurred and enlarged slowly.
>*n.* enlargement

enlarged *adj.* grown larger
>Enlarged lymph nodes.
>The heart was enlarged with normal arteries.

enough *adv.* sufficiently
>**enough** is rare in formal scientific English; **sufficiently** or **adequately** are more common.

enquire, inquire *vi. vt.* to seek information
>The questionnaire /enquired/simpler: asked/ about their age and mental status.
>In BE, **enquire** = to ask a question, **inquire** = to investigate: We /inquired into/investigated/studied/ this phenomenon.

enquiry, inquiry *n.* a request for information
>Door-to-door enquiry, postal enquiry.
>To make enquiries about = to ask questions about.

enrich *vt.* to increase the proportion of a desirable ingredient in
>To enrich a growth medium with nutrients.

enrol, enroll *vt.* to enter, register
>The study enrolled 20 patients = Twenty patients were enrolled in the study.
>*Compare*: include
>*n.* enrolment

enter *vt.*
>1. to come or go into
>Sensory fibres enter the spinal cord through the posterior roots.
>This acid enters red cells in an undissociated form.
>2. to become selected as a study subject

Ten patients entered the study.

Compare: enrol

entire *adj.* whole

The entire study period.

entity *n.* something with a separate independent existence

A disease entity = simpler: a disease.

A clinical entity = simpler: a disease.

entry *n.* the act of entering

The entry of infection into the bloodstream was from an extravascular focus.

The wound provided a portal of entry for the pathogen.

They were randomly allocated to two groups on entry /to/into/ the study.

This disease was present at /entry into the study/study entry/.

environment *n.* surroundings

The bacteria proliferated because of a favourable environment.

The ulcers provided a fertile environment for bacterial growth.

adj. environmental

episode *n.* an attack of a disease, a symptom

An episode of bleeding, coughing, cystitis, hypoglycaemia.

Overt, transient episodes of illness.

Compare: attack, bout, fit

episodic *adj.* occurring in episodes

Episodic ⟷ chronic forms of headache.

eponym *n.* a term derived from the name of a person, usually a research worker who was the first to describe the medical concept in question

Krebs cycle = citric acid cycle.

Paget's disease = osteitis deformans.

equal *adj.* identical or similar in size, number, value, rank, etc.

Equal amounts of substrate were used in the two experiments.

In a normal subject water intake is equal to water output.

equate *vt.* to regard as equal

Hypomagnesaemia is often equated with magnesium depletion.

equi-effective *adj.* equally effective

At equi-effective doses, fenoprofen causes less microbleeding than does aspirin.

equilibrium *n.* balance

To be in equilibrium.

Opposite: disequilibrium

equipotent *adj.* equally potent

An equipotent dose, drug.

equitoxic *adj.* equally toxic
A low-dose equitoxic treatment.
equivalence, equivalency *n.* the state or quality of being equivalent
The therapeutic equivalence of two drugs.
equivalent *adj.* having the same effect or value
65 mg codeine has been shown to be equivalent to about 60 mg aspirin.
Compare: equal
equivocal *adj.* subject to varying interpretations, uncertain
All patients had negative or equivocal treadmill tests.
Opposite: unequivocal
eradicate *vt.* to destroy or remove completely
This treatment eradicates bacteria from the intestine.
To eradicate convulsive seizures.
To /eradicate/extirpate/ a disease from a geographical area.
eradication *n.* removal
The eradication of a pathogenic agent, an infection, metastases.
erroneous *adj.* characterized by error, incorrect
Erroneous conclusions, diagnosis.
error *n.* a serious mistake; malfunction
Clerical errors may have catastrophic consequences.
Without laboratory confirmation, a clinical diagnosis of this disease is subject to error.
Inborn errors of metabolism.
Laboratory, ward errors.
Metabolic errors = metabolic disturbances.
escape *vt.* to manage to avoid (a disease)
To escape a disease.
essential *adj.*
1. vitally important
Peptic activity is not essential for protein digestion.
2. idiopathic
Essential hypertension.
establish *vt.* to prove
The role of these antibodies has not been established = It is still incompletely understood.
Tolerance to the drug was established from haematological studies.
To establish diagnosis, the cause of a disease.
Compare: confirm
established *adj.* widely accepted
Parenteral nutrition is an established method of feeding patients who are seriously ill.

estimate *vt.* to form a rough idea (of amount, size, intensity, etc.)

Sodium deficits may be estimated from a change in body weight.

The prevalence of lethal disease has been estimated at about 1/60 000 live births.

estimate *n.* appraisal

To /make an estimate of/estimate/ the degree of a burn.

According to cautious estimates.

estimation *n.* appraisal

We /made/undertook/ serum amylase estimations in all patients.

Compare: determination

et al. *abbr.* = and others (in referring to the authors of a study)

Brown *et al.*

Synonymous expressions: Brown and (his) associates, Brown and (his) colleagues, Brown and (his) co-workers

ethical *adj.* of morals

An ethical decision, problem.

The study was approved by the hospital /ethical/ethics/ committee.

evacuate *vt.* to discharge

To evacuate stools from the bowel.

evacuation *n.* removal

Evacuation of faeces, blood.

evaluable *adj.* assessable

The responses of these patients were not evaluable because of inadequate medical records.

evaluate *vt.* to assess, examine

The compound was evaluated for its ability to inhibit histamine release.

The patient was evaluated to determine the cause of her anaemia.

This test evaluates the severity of an asthma attack.

adj. evaluable

evaluation *n.* examination, assessment

A general medical evaluation.

Careful/meticulous/evaluation of a patient, of the family history.

Evaluation of the gastrointestinal tract showed marked malabsorption.

This treatment has undergone extensive clinical evaluation.

evanescent *adj.* disappearing, transient

Babies with evanescent heart murmurs.

Evanescent rash.

Compare: transient

event *n.* a condition occurring at a definite time

The risk of future cardiac events in these patients is related to the extent of myocardial ischaemia.

in the event of = plainly: in

In the event of/simply: in/ shock, there is a disadvantage in using both beta and alpha blockade.

eventual *adj.* ultimate

The management of these patients will depend on the eventual diagnosis.

adv. eventually = ultimately

evidence *n.* observations on which a conclusion can be based

To find, obtain evidence on the effects of smoking.

Offer, produce, provide, put forward, give evidence.

This evidence confirms, supports our previous findings.

This evidence indicates, shows, suggests that . . .

A growing body of evidence supports this contention.

This evidence favours our theory.

Evidence was /obtained/derived/ from observations . . .

Two patients had radiographic evidence of expansion of the gland.

Firm, strong, overwhelming evidence.

Consistent, convincing, experimental, irrefutable evidence.

Anecdotal evidence, conflicting, unconvincing evidence.

Evidence /for/in favour of/in support of/ ⟷ against a diagnosis.

evidence *vt.* to make evident

The infection was /evidenced/plainly: shown/ by persistent bacteriuria.

evident *adj.* easy to see or understand, readily apparent, clear because of evidence

Lymphopenia /is evident/plainly: occurs/ during active sarcoidosis.

These changes were evident in x-ray studies.

Synonymous or slightly different in meaning: **obvious** = easily evident; **apparent** = clearly seen or understood, but some reasoning may be required

evince *vt.* to evidence

Note: This is a rare verb, **show** has the same meaning.

evoke *vt.* (rare) to produce

Rising intracranial pressure may /evoke/simply: produce/ a rise in subarachnoid pressure.

Compare: produce

n. evocation

evolution *n.* gradual development

These cases generally have a slow evolution.

evolve *vi.* to develop gradually, to progress

As the disease evolved, mucopurulent expectoration developed.

The acute inflammatory process evolved into an abscess.

exacerbate *vt.* to make worse

The pain was exacerbated by movement.

Compare: aggravate, deteriorate, worsen

exacerbation *n.* worsening

Exacerbation of pain, symptoms, the clinical picture.

To relieve exacerbations.

Compare: aggravation, deterioration, worsening

Opposites: remission, improvement

exaggerated *adj.* abnormally increased or severe

His reflexes were exaggerated.

examination *n.* a physical inspection, a laboratory study of samples

To /carry out/make/ a physical examination, an x-ray examination.

Neurological examination /disclosed/showed/ distal sensory loss.

The examination showed a drowsy, disoriented man = On examination the man appeared drowsy and disoriented.

The disease can be /diagnosed/recognized/ on clinical examination.

examine *vt.* to scrutinize carefully

The kidneys were examined for /evidence/the presence/ of this disease.

The sample was examined histologically.

Compare: evaluate, explore, inspect

exceed *vt.* to be greater than

The concentration exceeded 80%.

excess *n.* an abnormally high amount or degree or the amount by which something exceeds

His food intake was in excess of body requirements.

Hypercalcaemia is usually due to excess breakdown of calcium.

Hormone excess ⟷ deficiency.

excess *adj.* abnormally high

Excess dietary calcium.

excessive *adj.* abnormally high

Excessive sodium intake.

exchange *n.* the act or action of exchanging

Gas exchange takes place in the lungs.

exchange *vt.* to give up one thing for another

The red cell membrane exchanges intracellular lithium ions for extracellular sodium ions.

Compare: replace, substitute

excise *vt.* to remove surgically

The tumour mass was excised after radical dissection.

n. excision

Compare: dissect

exclude *vt.*

1. to leave out

To /exclude/leave out/ a patient from a trial.

2. to rule out in diagnosis

Malaria was excluded by staining of blood films.

Opposite: include

exclusion *n.* the act or action of leaving or ruling out

The exclusion of a patient from a study ⟵⟶ admission to.

There are no specific tests for non-A non-B viruses and the diagnosis has to be based on exclusion.

excrete *vt.* to remove metabolic waste and end-products from the body

The drug is excreted unchanged in the urine.

Compare: secrete

excretion *n.* elimination from the body

The excretion of a substance by the kidneys.

excretory *adj.* pertaining to excretion

Impaired renal excretory function.

excruciating *adj.* very severe

Excruciating pain.

exercise *n.* physical exertion

Exercise rehabilitation, testing, training.

Bradycardia was assessed both at rest and during exercise.

His asthma was induced by exercise.

Vigorous exercise produces narrowing of the airways in most asthmatic patients.

Exercise-induced asthma.

exercise *vt.* to subject to physical exertion

To exercise a muscle.

exertion *n.* strenuous effort

Dyspnoea occurred /on exertion/during exercise/.

exertional *adj.* related to exertion

Exertional dyspnoea.

exertionally *adv.* by/on/exertion

Exertionally induced breathlessness.

exhaust *vt.* to use up completely

To exhaust body iron stores.

Compare: deplete

exhibit *vt.* to show, have

This verb is usually replaceable by **show** or **have**

To /exhibit/show/have/ normal plasma renin concentrations.

To /exhibit/show/have/ sensitivity to an allergen.

To /exhibit/show/have/ symptoms.

Compare: disclose, display, manifest, reveal, show

expand *vi. vt.* to increase in extent, surface or bulk

The lungs hold about 6 litres of air when expanded.

n. expansion

experience *n.* direct personal participation; accumulated knowledge

Experience has shown that . . .

Our initial, preliminary experience suggests this.

Our recent experience supports our previous report.

Our experience /in/with/ these patients is /encouraging/ favourable.

Our experience of this technique is limited.

In our experience this treatment is very effective.

experience *vt.* to have

They /experienced/plainly: had/ severe pain.

experienced *adj.* having experience

These doctors are experienced in cancer chemotherapy.

Opposite: inexperienced

experiment *n.* a test, an investigation, a trial

To /conduct/carry out//experiments on animals/animal experiments/.

experiment *vi.* to carry out experiments

To experiment with animals.

experimental *adj.* relating to an experiment

Experimental/laboratory/test/ animals.

The experimental group ⟷ the control group.

The drug is still in the experimental stage.

expert *adj.* skilful

To be expert /at/in/ cardiac surgery.

The operation carries no risk in expert hands.

expert *n.* a person with special skill or knowledge

He is an expert /at/in/ plastic surgery.

expire *vi.* to breathe out; to come to an end

Avoid **expire** as a euphemism for **die**.

explain *vt.* to make clear, to give or be the reason for

The purpose of the study was fully explained to the patients.

Compare: account for

explanation *n.* a statement that explains

A plausible explanation for this phenomenon /lies in/is/ the fact that . . .

explanatory *adj.* serving to explain

An explanatory note.

exploration *n.* surgical examination

A rewarding exploration of an organ.

exploratory *adj.* serving to explore

Exploratory laparotomy, surgery, thoracotomy.

explore *vt.* to examine, investigate

To explore an organ for signs of a disease.

explosive *adj.* very rapid or severe

Explosive diarrhoea.

The onset of this disease is explosive.

exponential *adj.* produced or expressed by multiplying a set of quantities by themselves

Exponential growth of bacteria.

exponentially *adv.* in an exponential fashion

The number of reported cases of this disease has risen exponentially (doubled annually).

expose *vt.*

1. to present to view

To expose tissues by dissection.

2. to make susceptible to

To be exposed to infection.

exposure *n.* the act or instance of exposing

Heavy ⟵⟶ light exposure.

They remained disabled despite exposure to numerous treatments.

To remove a patient from exposure to disease-inducing factors.

express *vt.*

1. to manifest

Follicular hyperplasia may be expressed clinically as lymphadenopathy.

2. to show in words or some other way

Nuclear volumes were expressed as percentages of the intracellular volume.

expression *n.* manifestation

Rickets and osteomalacia differ in their pathological expression.

This finding is /an expression/a sign/ of senile heart disease.

Compare: manifestation, sign

extend *vi. vt.*

    1. to (cause to) increase in size, to prolong

    To extend treatment /beyond (the time of)/after/ healing.

    2. to reach a certain point in distance, space or time

    The tip of the spleen extended to the iliac crest.

extension *n.*

    1. the act of extending, the state of being extended

    The extension of a patient's hospital stay.

    2. (an) increase in size or involvement

    The extension of a tumour beyond an organ.

    The extension of a virus infection into the central nervous system.

extensive *adj.* wide, far-reaching

    Extensive involvement, research.

extensively *adv.* widely

    Carcinoma of the bronchus is noted for its tendency to metastasize extensively.

extirpation *n.* eradication

    The extirpation of a disease.

    The /extirpation/complete removal/ of an organ.

    v. extirpate

extract *vt.*

    1. to pull out

    To extract a tooth.

    2. to take out by chemical means

    To extract a drug from the juice of a plant.

    n. extraction

extract *n.* the product of extraction

    Phytohaemagglutinin is an extract of the seeds of a bean plant.

extrapolate *vt.* to expand from known data into something not known

    One may extrapolate the results of this study to clinical practice.

    Compare: apply

    n. extrapolation

extremity *n.* limb

    Use plain words such as **ankle, arm, finger, foot, hand,** or **limb** instead of **extremity**

extrinsic *adj.* originating from the outside

    Haemolysis may be due to abnormalities extrinsic to the red blood cells.

    Opposite: intrinsic

extrude *vi. vt.* to press out, to (cause to) protrude
The sodium pump extrudes sodium out of the cell.
An extruding tooth had migrated from its socket.
n. extrusion

F

fabricate *vt.* to invent

    To fabricate an illness.

    n. fabrication

facilitate *vt.* to make easy or easier

    This position will facilitate coughing.

    n. facilitation

facility *n.* means, equipment

    Facilities for intubation were readily available and the patient survived.

    A hospital with surgical facilities.

factor *n.* an agent or element that actively contributes to a result

    Age is an important risk factor for ischaemic heart disease.

failure *n.*

    1. severe insufficiency, incompetence

    Management, correction of circulatory failure.

    Patients with heart failure.

    Visual failure due to optic nerve atrophy.

    Compare: compromise, decompensation, embarrassment, insufficiency

    2. unsuccessful effort

    Failure to visualize the biliary tree delayed the diagnosis.

    Treatment failure.

fall *n.*

    1. a decrease

    Administration of lactose resulted in a fall in faecal calcium.

    Opposite: rise

    2. a sudden descent

    A fall from a height.

fall *vi.* to decrease

    The creatinine clearance fell below 10 ml/min.

    The mortality and morbidity of this disease have fallen substantially.

    Opposite: rise

    Compare: decline, decrease

fall-off *n.* decline in quantity

    A /fall-off/fall/ in established urine output.

false *adj.* not in accordance with the true condition

    A false-negative test shows a negative reaction, even if disease is present and a false-positive test shows a positive reaction, even if disease is absent.

A false reading.
Compare: spurious
Opposite: true

familial *adj.* relating to the family
The familial occurrence of sleep-walking.

family history *n.* *See*: history

family study *n.* investigation of a family
Family studies have suggested that this disease is hereditary.

fare *vi.* to get on, progress
These patients /fared/did/ better than those treated by bypass.

fast *n.* a period of fasting
The study was carried out after an overnight fast.

fast *vi. vt.* to (cause to) abstain from eating
The results were obtained in /subjects who had fasted/fasting subjects/.
Patients in the fasting state.

fatal *adj.* causing death
The disease is fatal, often because of respiratory complications.

fatality *n.* a death
Fatalities due to hyperkalaemia are rare.

fate *n.*
1. the final stages of metabolism
The fate of this lipid is unclear, but it is probably removed by the liver.
2. outcome
The fate of children with Huntington's chorea may be unknown until they are well into child-bearing age.

fatig(u)ability *n.* susceptibility to tiredness
Easy, undue fatiguability is a common subjective symptom of heart failure

fatigue *n.* tiredness
Fatigue was reported in 50% of the study subjects.
Postoperative fatigue.

favour (BE), **favor** (AE)
1. *vt.* to support
This sign favoured the diagnosis of a cholestatic over a hepatocellular process.
2. *n.* acceptance
Digoxin has found favour in the treatment of heart disease.
This theory has been abandoned in favour of a new better one.
This treatment has fallen out of favour.

favourable (BE), **favorable** (AE) *adj.* advantageous
A favourable response was obtained with this treatment.

feasible *adj.* practicable
A feasible treatment programme.
feature *n.* a distinctive part or quality
The clinical features of a disease (=its signs and symptoms).
The distinguishing features of a disease.
The radiological features of a cyst.
febrile *adj.* of or caused by fever
A febrile patient; febrile convulsions; the number of febrile days.
Opposite: afebrile
feed *vt.* to give food
The patient was fed by nasogastric tube.
feedback *n.* the flow of information from a later phase of a process to an earlier phase (WHO 1)
The pituitary control of the thyroid incorporates a feedback loop so that plasma TSH tends to increase as thyroid hormone concentration falls and vice versa.
feeding *n.*
1. the giving of food
Breast, intravenous, nasogastric feeding.
2. a meal
Frequent small feedings are preferred to three large meals.
female *n.* a woman or, generally, the sex that produces gametes (egg cells) to be fertilized by male sperm.
It has been suggested that **a female** should not be used as a synonym of **a woman patient** or **a woman subject**.
The study included 10 men and 15 women (instead of: 10 males and 15 females)
female can be used as an attribute: a female patient
Girls and women collectively = females
adj. female
few *adj.* not many
Few/only a few/ patients were satisfied with this treatment.
film *n.*
1. a thin layer of any material
Films of peripheral blood were made on methanol-cleaned glass coverslips.
2. photography material
A chest film = a chest radiograph.
Findings on an x-ray film.
find *vt.* to discover
We found that his negative nitrogen balance was due to protein loss.
They were found to have osteoarthropathy.

Compare: discover, encounter

finding *n.* the result of investigation or observation

A /chance/fortuitous/incidental/, clinical, experimental finding.

A finding may be overlooked or ignored.

Findings on liver biopsy.

fine *adj.*

1. very pure

Fine chemicals.

2. relating to the smallest details

The fine structure of human embryo development.

3. delicate

A fine ($\longleftrightarrow$ coarse) tremor occurred on physical exertion.

firm *adj.* solid, hard

The lesion was firm to palpation.

first-degree relatives *n.* parents, sib(ling)s and children

fit *n.* a sudden attack

A grand mal fit (in epilepsy).

fit *adj.* in good health

He was medically fit for work.

The patient was a fit 36-year-old man.

flare-up *n.* a sudden intensification, reactivation

Flare-ups of tinea occur more often during the summer.

Resumption of smoking may cause a flare-up of thrombo-angitis.

flare up *vi.* to intensify suddenly, reactivate

The arthritis flared up and produced fresh symptoms.

flitting *adj.* moving rapidly from one site to another in the body

Flitting arthritis.

florid *adj.* fully developed

He had florid skeletal stigmata of Marfan's syndrome.

Florid cirrhosis.

fluctuate *vi.* to rise and fall

The fever, pain fluctuated in intensity.

Compare: oscillate, swing

fluctuation *n.* a variation, undulation

Fluctuations in the course of a disease = remissions and exacerbations.

Compare: oscillation, swing

flush *n.* reddening

A persistent flush of the skin.

flush *vi. vt.*

1. *vt.* to cleanse with a liquid

The kidney was preserved by cold flushing with a hyper-osmolar solution.

2. *vi. vt.* to (cause to) become red

Her cheeks were flushed with fever.

focal *adj.* limited to a specific part of the body

A focal disease process.

(In epilepsy:) focal seizures ⟷ generalized seizures.

focus *n.* (pl. **foci, focuses**) the centre of a disease process

A disease focus.

A focus of inflammation.

focus *vt.* to concentrate

The study focussed (AE focussed) on two problems.

To focus a study on a phenomenon.

To focus one's attention on.

following *prep.* after

Plasma concentrations were measured following a single dose of the drug.

follow-through *n.* observation of the passage of a substance through the body

An obstruction of the small intestine was seen on barium meal and follow-through.

follow-up *n.* re-examination of a patient at intervals

To carry out a follow-up.

Benefits of the treatment were seen at long-term follow-up.

He failed to return for follow-up.

Colonoscopy may be done on follow-up.

Relapses were seen on follow-up.

They were lost to follow-up because they refused to participate in the study or moved from the area.

follow up, follow *vt.* to maintain contact with a patient to assess the effectiveness of a treatment

He was /followed up/followed/ as an outpatient at regular intervals with pulmonary function tests.

follow-up phase *n.* the period of follow-up

He entered a three-month follow-up phase.

follow-up visit *n.* a follow-up session

Blood pressure was measured at each follow-up visit.

To make a follow-up visit.

food *n.* a substance supplied as nourishment

Food and fluid were allowed only three hours after administration of the drug.

for *prep.*

1. expressing purpose

The child was accepted for admission.

The drug was prescribed for obesity.

2. expressing the purpose of finding

The patient was examined, diagnosed, monitored, observed, screened, tested for signs or symptoms of a disease.

The liver was studied for (the presence of) these signs.

The lungs were auscultated for rales.

3. in regard to, with regard to, as regards

He was oriented for time and place.

Spinal fluid was negative for the antigen.

The changes in each variable for each patient were calculated.

foreign *adj.* coming from without

Foreign bodies in the nose are common in young children.

To retrieve a foreign body from the bladder.

Compare: extrinsic

forestall *vt.* to prevent beforehand

Careful observation will forestall increased loss of scleral substance.

foretell *vt.* to signify

Decreased hearing acuity may foretell more serious side-effects.

Compare: herald, precede

form *n.*

1. the external features, shape and size of a structure

2. a standardized document with spaces for insertion of required information

A standarized case-record form.

An informed-consent form.

form *vi. vt.* to (cause to) be produced, to develop

In the dog very little acid forms after administration of salicylate.

Metabolites /form/are formed/ in synthetic reactions.

n. formation

fortify *vt.* to increase the nutritional value of a food

The bread was fortified with ferrous salts.

Compare: enrich

fortuitous *adj.* occurring sporadically

This is a fortuitous complication in patients undergoing vagotomy.

Compare: incidental

frank *adj.* clinically evident

Frank congestive heart failure.

Frank oedema, frank symptoms of acute schizophrenia.

free *adj.*

1. chemically uncombined

Free nitrogen.
2. from = without, lacking
Free from symptoms.
Low dosage treatment may be free from this risk.
3. free of = not affected by, not dependent on
Free of alcohol and drugs.
Compound adjectives: disease-free, drug-free, symptom-free
freedom *n.* the quality or state of being free
Freedom from residual live virus.
They claimed total freedom from headache after surgery.
frequency *n.*
1. the rate of occurrence per unit of time or population
Resistant viruses arose at a high frequency.
2. frequent micturition.
Diurnal frequency; night frequency.
frequent *adj.* common
This is a frequent finding in preterm babies.
Opposites: infrequent, rare
from *prep.*
1. expressing the source or origin
To obtain information from the white cell count.
Studies from Seattle have shown that . . .
2. expressing the cause (=due to, owing to)
Central nervous system depression from drugs.
Mortality from a disease.
The eye was blind from atrophy of the optic nerve head.
The joint was swollen from bony overgrowth.
3. expressing the basis of something with verbs such as /appear/
seem/, calculate, conclude, deduce, describe, diagnose, judge
From these findings it appears that . . .
fruitless *adj.* unproductive
A fruitless examination, search
Compare: disappointing, frustrating, unrewarding
frustrating *adj.* disappointing
Recurrent bronchogenic carcinoma remains a frustrating disease to the oncologist.
full *adj.*
1. filled to capacity
A full bladder.
2. not limited
All his joint movements were full.
full-blown *adj.* fully developed
Full-blown encephalopathy may be precipitated by sedatives.
Compare: florid

fulminant *adj.* sudden and severe

Episodes of fulminant, often lethal, bacterial infection occurred.

Fulminant hepatic failure.

fulminating *adj.* fulminant

Most bacterial brain abscesses have an acute fulminating course.

function *n.*

1. the natural action (of an organ)

Auditory, visual function.

Pulmonary function; ventilatory function of the lungs.

The kidney /exerts/simply: has/ an important antihypertensive function.

2. a factor dependent on another factor

The level of body iron stores is a function of dietary intake and intestinal iron absorption.

v. function

functional *adj.*

1. pertaining to function

Functional disturbances.

2. functioning properly

His kidneys were functional.

fund *vt.* to provide funds or money

This study was funded in part by a donation.

further *adj.* additional

A further seven specimens will be required.

This hypothesis deserves further investigation.

future *n.* the time after the present

The future holds many exciting possibilities.

The future will show if this theory is correct.

G

gain *n.* increase
Weight gain.

gain *vi. vt.*
1. *vi.* to increase, advance
This operation is gaining in popularity.
To gain weight.
2. *vt.* to obtain (more of)
To gain experience, to gain data from examinations.

general *adj.*
1. relating to the whole body, systemic
General ⟷ regional, local anaesthesia.
2. treating all illnesses, not specializing
A general hospital, general practice; a general practitioner.

generalized, generalised *adj.* not restricted to a particular area of the body
A generalized infection spread throughout the body or changed from a localized infection to a systemic one.
Opposite: localized/localised

generally *adv.* usually
Patients given a prosthetic valve are generally believed to require lifelong anticoagulants.

generic *adj.*
1. general, shared by a whole class of things
Gastroenteritis is a generic term, often implying a non-specific, uncertain or unknown cause.
Opposite: specific
2. not protected by a trademark, non-proprietary
Paracetamol is the generic term for the drug that is sold under several /brand/proprietary/trade/ names.
A generic drug ⟷ a proprietary drug.

generous *adj.* containing a large amount
Generous biopsy specimens were obtained.

gently *adv.* not violently or excessively
Shake gently!
This solution should be warmed gently.

germ *n.* a pathogenic microorganism
Note: **germ** is rare in scientific papers

gestation *n.* the period of development of the embryo in viviparous animals between conception and birth
Compare: pregnancy

gestational *adj.* pertaining to gestation
The baby was small for gestational age.
give *vt.*
1. to administer
To give a drug by injection.
The drug was given intravenously at a dosage of 200 mg a day in these patients.
2. to cause
Intravenous injection gave stronger analgesia.
give rise to *v.* to cause
The drug may give rise to potentially fatal arrhythmias.
given *adj.* receiving
Patients given this drug.
global *adj.* comprehensive
Global and regional abnormalities of ventricular function.
Global dementia = dementia affecting all cognitive functions and skills.
He had global muscle wasting.
go *vi.* to pass
The attack went unnoticed.
goal *n.* a specific state towards which actions and resources are directed. Unlike objectives and targets, goals are not constrained by time or existing resources, nor are they necessarily attainable, but are rather an ultimate desired state towards which actions and resources are directed (WHO 1)
Unloading the heart from the double burden of obesity and hypertension should become the major goal of preventive cardiology.
govern *vt.* to control
The concentration of renin is governed by the kidney.
Compare: control, modulate, regulate
grade *n.* degree
Low-grade fever.
grade *vt.* to classify, categorize
Each patient was graded for the maximal severity of the disease during the episode.
The pain was graded as severe in 10% of patients.
gradual *adj.* occurring or developing by steps or degrees
A gradual decline in health.
gradually *adv.* by steps or degrees, slowly
The patient recovered gradually.
gratifying *adj.* satisfactory, pleasing
Treatment was gratifying since marked regression of the skin lesions occurred.

Compare: encouraging, rewarding

grave *adj.* serious

This disease has a grave outlook.

gravid *adj.* pregnant

The gravid uterus may displace a cardiac catheter by raising the diaphragm.

Note: In other contexts, **pregnant** is the usual English word.

gross *adj.*

1. marked, conspicuous

Gross abnormality, deficiency, haemorrhage, malnutrition, oedema, oversimplification.

2. rough, showing general aspects without fine distinctions

A gross estimation of blood flow.

The gross appearance of the sputum is not diagnostic in streptococcal pneumonia.

adv. grossly

grounds *n.* basis, reason

She was advised against pregnancy on medical grounds.

There were strong grounds for believing that the disease was caused by a virus.

They were divided into three groups on clinical grounds.

on the grounds that = simply: because

group *n.* a number of people (patients) with some unifying common factor

To allocate, assign, categorize, divide into groups.

To fall, fit into groups.

group *vt.* to divide into groups

These drugs are grouped into five categories.

grow *vi. vt.*

1. *vt.* to cultivate, culture

This virus can be grown in tissue culture.

2. *vi.* to increase in size, develop

Nerve cells are difficult to grow in culture.

The lung mass had grown slowly over a period of 15 years.

growth *n.*

1. increase in size, development

Human growth.

2. tumour

The malignant growth was excised.

guarding *n.* protection against possible pain

There was mild, diffuse tenderness to deep abdominal palpation, with voluntary guarding.

guidance *n.* help, advice

We were given expert guidance /on/with/ the interpretation of these biopsy findings.

guide *vt.* to direct the movement or course of

Ultrasound is used to guide the biopsy needle to these lesions.

guide *n.* something that provides guiding information

Plasma osmolality is an accurate guide to intracellular osmolality.

Compare: index, indicator, marker

guideline *n.* a standard or criterion of subsequent measures

There are well-defined guidelines for preventing the transmission of this disease.

H

habituation *n.* drug habituation = drug dependence

hallmark *n.* a distinguishing feature

Striking transaminase elevations are the hallmark of acute viral hepatitis.

hand *n.*

Atropine should always be /on hand/readily available/ for these acute attacks.

close at hand = readily, immediately available

handicap *n.* a disadvantage for a given individual resulting from an impairment or a disability, that limits or prevents the fulfilment of a role that is normal (depending on age, sex, and social and cultural factors) for that individual (WHO 2).

Disease, disorder /impairment/disability/handicap (WHO 2)

A hearing handicap, a social integration handicap.

handicapped *adj.* suffering from a handicap

Aurally handicapped; handicapped by diabetes.

handle *vt.*

1. to treat

Heart failure was /handled/treated/ by administering digitalis.

2. to tolerate

The elderly /handle/tolerate/ rifampicin poorly.

handling *n.* processing

The renal handling of urea.

hangover *n.* after effects (of alcohol or a drug)

They complained of hangover with diazepam.

harbour (BE), **harbor** (AE) *vt.* to have, contain (often: a pathogen)

Bed linen used by a patient was found to harbour the bacteria.

harbinger *n.* something that foretells something else

His cytomegalovirus infection was a harbinger of AIDS.

hard *adj.* not easy to penetrate

The entire ischiorectal fossa was replaced by woody hard tissue.

Opposite: soft

harm *n.* injury

To do harm to.

vt. harm

harmful *adj.* injurious

Harmful bacteria.

Opposites: harmless, innocent

have *vt*.
1. to obtain
He had abnormal pulmonary function studies.
2. to undergo
Two patients had had a gastrectomy = They had a history of gastrectomy.
3. to suffer from
She had malabsorption of carbohydrate.

hazard *n*. a risk
Dust is an occupational hazard.
Environmental hazards.
Obesity is a /hazard to health/health hazard/.
This treatment has many potential hazards.

hazardous *adj*. involving a risk
A hazardous method, occupation.

heal *vi*. *vt*. to (cause to) become well or healthy
Pulmonary infarcts may heal by absorption.
The lesion healed without surgery, with scarring.

health *n*. the general condition of the body
He had bad health = He suffered ill health.
He was in full, good ⟷ poor health.
The pH of extracellular fluid in /health/a healthy subject/ is maintained at about 7.4.

healthy *adj*.
1. enjoying health
Healthy volunteers.
She delivered a healthy girl.
2. good for health
A healthy climate.

heavy *adj*. excessive
Heavy drinking, smoking.

helpful *adj*. useful
This drug is helpful in (controlling) diarrhoea.
This sign is helpful in making the diagnosis.
Compare: beneficial, useful, valuable

helpfulness *n*. usefulness
The degree of helpfulness of the treatment was related to dose.
Compare: benefit, value

herald *vt*. to precede
The termination of these attacks were heralded by pronounced coughing.
Compare: announce, precede

hereditary *adj*. transmitted genetically
A hereditary disease.

heredity *n.* the genetic transmission of biological factors from one generation to another
Some diseases are due to environmental factors, others are due to heredity.

heroic *adj.* highly intense
Despite /heroic measures/massive effort/, the patient died.

high *adj.* greater than normal in degree, amount, etc.
High carbon dioxide mixtures.
His diet was high in fibre = He had a high-fibre diet.
Compare: rich

high-dose *adj.* with large doses
High-dose treatment.
Note: low-dose, medium-dose, moderate-dose

high-grade *adj.* severe, serious
High-grade fever; high-grade biliary obstruction.

highlight *vt.* to draw attention to
The study highlighted some shortcomings of this treatment.

high-risk *adj. see*: risk

highly *adv.* to a high degree
A highly significant number of virus infections.
Cerebral tumours are highly invasive.

hinder *vt.* to prevent
Standard therapeutic approaches are hindered by late discovery of ovarian carcinoma.
Compare: forestall, preclude, prevent

historical *adj.* pertaining to a case history
A meticulous historical search was made for environmental clues to specific antigen exposure.

history *n.* the patient's medical background and story
A man with a 24-hour history of vomiting.
The patient gives, has, presents with a history; the physician discovers, elicits, finds, obtains, takes the history.
An accurate, detailed, relevant, unremarkable history.
She had no antecedent medical history, no antibiotic history.
She had no history of having taken any antibiotics.
A longstanding, recent history of diarrhoea; a regular menstrual history.
Diabetes was suspected from the history.

history; family history *n.* the clinical status and medical history of the members of the patient's family
A positive family history of diabetes was found.
There was a /clear/strong/ family history of diabetes running through several generations.
Opposite: personal history

history; natural history of a disease = its usual course and features

history; past history (PH) of a patient = his medical history before present illness = antecendent, previous history

hold *vt.* to believe

It has been generally held that growth retardation in congenital rubella is not due to a disturbance of endocrine function.

home *n.* the place where one lives

The patient's home circumstances.

Home dialysis.

Home visits by doctors.

Accidents in the home.

adj. domiciliary

hospital *n.* a residential establishment providing short-term and long-term medical care. In BE, unlike in AE, **hospital** is used without any article, when it refers to hospital treatment, not the building(s):

Delivery in hospital ⟷ at home.

He died in hospital (BE), in the hospital (AE).

To admit a patient (to hospital) ⟷ to discharge.

To take a patient to hospital (BE), to the hospital (AE).

Babies born at this hospital.

Hospital practice ⟷ general practice.

Under strictly controlled hospital conditions.

Hospital-based studies ⟷ community-based studies.

Hospital controls ⟷ controls selected from the community.

Hospital patients ⟷ general practice patients, domiciliary patients.

This is a 500-bed public acute-care teaching hospital serving the population of Beek County.

hospital-acquired *adj.* acquired during hospital stay

Serious hospital-acquired infections are caused by Gram-negative rods.

hospital-based *adj.* based at a hospital

Hospital-based respiratory therapy.

hospitalization *n.* (AE) hospital admission, treatment or stay

They required hospitalization for further evaluation.

To die /during hospitalization (AE)/in hospital (BE).

hospitalize (AE) *vt.* = (BE) admit (to hospital)

He was hospitalized with hypertension.

Compare: to rehospitalize = readmit

host *n.* the person or animal harbouring a disease or a parasite

Host responses to infection.

The effect of a malignant tumour on the host.

hourly *adj.* occurring hour by hour, given every hour

The ulcer patient was given /hourly antacids/antacids hourly/.
adv. hourly

human *adj.* relating to man
Human milk.

human *n.* man, a human being
Pituitary glands of the human, horse and chicken were studied.
The drug is well tolerated in /humans/man.

hypersensitive *adj.* abnormally sensitive (to an allergen)
Hypersensitive to cold, to pollen.
n. hypersensitivity

hypothesis *n.* an idea which serves as a starting-point of reasoning
or explanation
To /advance/form/put forth/put forward/ a hypothesis.
To base a hypothesis on findings.
To confirm, support a hypothesis.
A tenable ⟷ untenable hypothesis.
adj. hypothetical

hypothesize, hypothesise *vt.* to form a hypothesis
Suggest or **take a view** are more common.
Compare: postulate

iceberg; the tip of an iceberg is a medical problem which is much larger than is first assumed

The number of AIDS patients discovered so far is merely the tip of an iceberg.

identical *adj.* exactly alike

A is identical /with/to/ B.

Placebo tablets of identical appearance.

Similar, but not identical.

identify *vt.* to recognize

These antigens are identified by their effects *in vitro*.

Ultrasound can identify the shape of the kidneys.

ill *adj.*.

1. sick, unwell

Critically, gravely, seriously, severely ill patients.

Ill with a disease.

2. adverse

The ill effects of bacteria on the normal bowel flora.

ill-advised *adj.* showing lack of sufficient consideration

An ill-advised operation.

ill-defined *adj.* poorly defined, vague

An ill-defined ($\longleftrightarrow$ well-marginated) patchy density was visible in the left lung.

The signs and symptoms of a disease may be ill-defined.

ill health *n.* illness

He suffered from ill health after an attack of acute mononucleosis.

illness *n.* an unhealthy state of the body

Illness is a state of ill health caused by a disease.

Unlike a disease, illness is not contagious or transmitted.

Compare: ailment, disease, disorder, sickness

ill-understood *adj.* not fully understood

The mechanism of this intoxication is ill-understood.

illustrate *vt.* to show

Fig. 1 illustrates lying and standing blood pressures.

adj. illustrative

n. illustration

image *n.*

1. a visual reproduction

To generate ultrasonic images.

2. a mental picture

A patient's /image of self/self-image/.

image *vt.* to produce an image

Imaging for the radiologist in a small hospital involves diagnostic x-ray work or ultrasound or both.

imbalance *n.* a lack of equilibrium, disequilibrium

A ventilation–perfusion imbalance leads to hypoxaemia.

An imbalance in the distribution of prognostic factors between study groups.

Compare: disequilibrium

immediate *adj.* direct in effect

The immediate effects on heart rate and blood pressure of withdrawing antihypertensive drugs

immediately *adv.* directly

They received the placebo immediately before the start of the study.

immune *adj.*

1. not susceptible

Such a patient is immune to the complications of hypertension.

2. protected by antibodies to an antigen

It should be ensured that all women of child-bearing age are immune to rubella.

3. another word for immunological(ly)

An immune response, immune competent, immune suppressed.

immunity *n.* ability to resist a disease

To establish, induce immunity in an individual to an antigen.

To /give/ confer/ immunity to an individual with a vaccine.

immunocompromised *adj.* immunologically weakened

Immunocompromised patients, especially those with a T-lymphoctye deficiency.

Compare: immunosuppressed ⟷ immunologically normal

impact *n.* an impelling effect

The impact of ageing on nutritional requirements.

Compare: effect, influence

impair *vt.* to damage, weaken

The drug may impair mental and/or physical abilities.

n. impairment

Compare: compromise, weaken

impaired *adj.* suffering from an impairment

Hearing-impaired/aurally handicapped/ subjects.

Mentally impaired old people, seriously impaired renal function.

impairment *n.* any loss or abnormality of psychological, physiological, or anatomical structure or function (WHO 2)

Intellectual, speech, visual impairment.

impart *vt.* to give

The right ventricle may impart an impulse to the fingertips.

impending *adj.* about to happen

Impending shock.

Compare: imminent

imperative *adj.* urgent

Isolation of these patients is imperative.

Compare: mandatory

impermeable *adj.* impenetrable, impervious

These parts of the nephron are impermeable to water.

impetus *n.* an incentive, a stimulus

The limitations of the present control methods have given a further impetus to work on the immunology of malaria.

impinge *vi.* to have an effect on

These lesions impinge on the gyrus of the temporal lobe.

implant *n.* something implanted

implant *vt.* to insert a tissue or an object into the body

The rods were implanted by needle into the pituitary gland.

To implant a pacemaker.

Compare: insert, introduce

adj. implanted, indwelling

n. implantation

implicate *vt.* to show to be involved

Cyclizine has been implicated as a teratogenic agent in animals.

Compare: incriminate

implication *n.* a(n indirect) consequence

These findings have important therapeutic implications.

v. imply

import *vt.* to bring in from an outside source

To import a disease from an endemic area.

n. importation

impression *n.* a mark left by pressing

An impression on the trachea made by a goitre.

improve *vi. vt.* to (cause to) become better

Radiotherapy improved the survival of these patients.

Their symptoms (were) improved by treatment.

They were improved with oxygen administration.

Improved methods, improved vital signs.

Compare: ameliorate, enhance, settle, subside

Opposites: deteriorate, exacerbate, weaken, worsen

improvement *n.* the act of improving, the state of being improved

He /had/showed / marked improvement

Improvement in a disease, mortality, prognosis, symptoms.

Improvement occurred on previous values.

Improvement was obtained with the treatment = The treatment produced improvement.

Compare: amelioration, enhancement, involution, subsidence

Opposites: deterioration, exacerbation, worsening

in *prep*.

1. expressing place, position

He is in hospital with severe anaemia.

Compare: He works at the hospital.

This finding occurred in patients with hypertension.

2. expressing condition

He was admitted in coma, shock, terminal renal failure.

Such inhibitors have been described /in pregnancy/in pregnant women//in health/in healthy subjects/.

This cardiac patient was in sinus rhythm.

inability *n*. lack of ability

Renal tubular acidosis is an inability to excrete an acid urine.

inaccessible *adj*. not capable of being reached

The lesions were inaccessible to surgery.

The duration of this treatment was inadequate.

n. inadequacy

inactive *adj*. quiescent

Inactive liver disease.

Compare: dormant, quiescent, silent

inapparent *adj*. not apparent

Clinically inapparent melioidosis may be latent for years.

Opposite: overt

inappropriate *adj*. not consistent with, unsuitable

His weight was inappropriate for his estimated gestational age.

Compare: disproportionate

inappropriately *adv*. inconsistently, unsuitably

Blood glucose concentrations are inappropriately high in diabetes mellitus.

inborn *adj*. present from birth

Inborn /genetically determined/ errors of metabolism.

Compare: congenital

incapable *adj*. unable

These cells are incapable of differentiating.

incapacitate *vt*. to deprive of strength

These violent seizures incapacitate the patient.

incapacitating *adj*. disabling

An incapacitating illness.

Compare: crippling, incapacitating

inception *n*. beginning

Some cancers are capable of metastasizing almost from their inception.

incidence *n.*

1. the rate of occurrence in a given period and population
The high ⟷ low incidence of a disease.
The incidence of side-effects is about 10% with this drug.

2. the number of instances of illness commencing, or of persons falling ill, during a given period in a specified population (WHO 1)
To reduce the incidence of a disease.
Compare: prevalence

incidental *adj.*

1. occurring in connection with a more important event
Intracranial haemorrhage incidental to birth trauma.
Splenectomy incidental to a peptic ulcer operation.

2. occurring merely by chance
An incidental finding.
Compare: fortuitous

incipient *adj.* beginning, at an early stage
Incipient cancer.

incision *n.* the act of cutting; a cut wound
The kidney was removed through a transverse abdominal incision.
v. incise

incite *vt.* to cause
This neoplasm may incite myositis.
Compare: cause, induce, produce

include *vt.* to admit
To include patients in a trial.
Opposite: exclude from
Compare: accept, admit, enrol, enter

inclusion *n.* the act or result of including
Ten patients were eligible for inclusion in the study
Opposite: exclusion (from a study)
Compare: admission, enrolment, entry

incompatible *adj.* incapable of being combined
An incompatible drug cannot be administered in combination with another drug.
Incompatible blood cannot be transfused.
n. incompatibility

incompetence *n.* physical or mental insufficiency
Mitral valve incompetence.
Compare: failure, insufficiency

incompetent *adj.* characterized by incompetence

Incompetent valves = leaky valves.

incompletely *adj.* not fully

This phenomenon remains incompletely explained.

inconclusive *adj.* not leading to a conclusion

The results of this study were inconclusive.

inconsistent *adj.* not consistent

This finding is inconsistent with the results of previous studies.

Compare: agreement

incontinent *adj.* relating to involuntary urination or defaecation.

She was incontinent of urine.

n. faecal/urinary incontinence

incorporate *vi. vt.* to include or be included

The drug is incorporated into the DNA of cancer cells.

increase *vi. vt.* to make or become greater (in size, amount or intensity)

The mortality rate increased with age.

Verbs such as *increase, decrease, reduce, and diminish* are often used in the passive to refer to body processes.

The relative volume of vascular elements was increased.

To increase /a food in nutritive value/the nutritive value of a food/.

Compare: add, augment, boost, build up, compound, step up

increase *n.* the act, process or result of increasing

A great, large ⟷ slight, small increase

increased *adj.*

If no change is being indicated, use **higher, commoner**.

An increased risk, a higher risk

increment *n.* increase

Stepwise increments of the dose.

adj. incremental

Opposite: decrement

incriminate *vt.* implicate

A virus has been incriminated /in/ as a cause of/ thyroiditis.

Compare: implicate

incur *vt.* to become subject to

They had incurred injuries in sports.

To incur pain

Compare: sustain

incurable *adj.* that cannot be cured

An incurable disease.

independent *adj.* not dependent

The effect was independent of treatment duration.

independent of ⟷ dependent on

index *n.* (*pl.* **indexes/indices**) a sign, indicator

Early diagnosis of this disease requires a high index of suspicion.

Improvement occurred in the indices of inflammatory joint activity.

This test /is/provides/ a sensitive index /of/for monitoring/ renal function.

indicate *vt.*

1. to be a sign or symptom of

Petit mal attacks rarely indicate gross brain damage.

These findings indicate that he was suffering from porphyria.

Compare: suggest

2. to recommend, require

Surgery was indicated in ten patients.

The drug is strongly indicated for (the treatment of) this disease.

Indicated /for/in/ children.

Opposite: contraindicate

indication *n.*

1. a sign pointing to the cause

These signs may be an early indication of serious blood disorders.

2. a sign that points to or serves as a guide to treatment

Clearer indications for surgery are needed in this case.

3. a condition for which a particular treatment is recommended

The indication for this drug is myasthenia gravis.

Opposite: contraindication

indicative *adj.* serving as a sign or guide

Ratios of urinary concentrations of oestriol might be indicative of cancer risk.

Indicative but not definitive.

indirect *adj.* not direct, with something between

An indirect symptom is indirectly due to the disease.

indiscriminate *adj.* lacking careful consideration

Indiscriminate use of antimicrobial drugs.

indistinguishable *adj.* very similar to

The clinical features of the disease may be indistinguishable from those of viral hepatitis.

individualize, individualise *vt.* to modify according to the requirements of an individual patient

The dosage of the drug must be individualized.

individual *adj.* relating to a single subject

The duration of an illness may vary considerably with the individual patient.

The individual requirements of a patient = the requirements of the individual patient.

indolent *adj.* causing little pain, slowly growing
An indolent tumour.
Subacute myelomonocytic leukaemia is an indolent disorder.

induce *vt.*
1. to cause
Ischaemia induces pain in skeletal muscles.
Lymphokine induces other lymphocytes to undergo transformation into lymphoblasts.
The drug induces gastrointestinal irritation.
To /induce reduction in /reduce/ mortality.
An experimentally induced disease.
Exercise-induced ischaemia = exercise ischaemia.
Induced ⟷ spontaneous abortion.
Compare: cause, produce
2. to initiate
The patient was induced into remission with a drug.
3. to induce anaesthesia
The patient was induced with thiopental.

inducer *n.* something that induces, an activator
Rifampicin is an inducer of hepatic drug metabolizing enzymes.

induction *n.* initiation
The artificial induction of labour.
The induction of anaesthesia.
The induction of renal lesions by a pathogen.
This factor is implicated in the induction of renal lesions.
Induction chemotherapy = chemotherapy as initial treatment before surgery or radiotherapy.

induration *n.* a hardened area
Skin indurations.
v. indurate

indwelling *adj.* implanted
An indwelling catheter.
Venous blood samples were obtained through an indwelling needle.

inebriated *adj.* (euphemistic usage:) intoxicated
n. inebriation

ineffective *adj.* that does not produce the desired effect
An ineffective treatment.

ineffectual *adj.* without the desired effect
ineffectual respiratory movements.

inept *adj.* incompetent, inappropriate

Inept needle manipulation.

Opposite: expert

inevitable *adj.* inescapable

This was an inevitable consequences of a radical operation.

inevitably *adv.* inescapably

Problems inevitably arise in continuing anticoagulant prophylaxis during pregnancy.

inexplicable *adj.* unexplained

Inexplicable headaches.

infancy *n.* the period from the end of the newborn period (1–4 weeks of life) to the assumption of the erect posture (12–14 months)

infant *n.* a young child; baby

infarct *n.* an area of dead tissue caused by obstructed blood flow to that tissue, usually as a complication of embolism

infarction *n.*

1. an infarct
2. the formation of an infarct

infect *vt.* to cause infection

Patients infected with this disease.

Systemic candidiasis may infect the kidney.

infection *n.* invasion of microorganisms in body tissues or infectious disease

Infection by direct contact.

Direct infection of the pelvis from the alimentary tract.

Infection from an organism, via the bloodstream.

Infection with poliovirus.

The symptoms begin about 5 days after infection.

adj. infectious

Compare: inflammation

infectious *adj.* caused by or causing a transmittable disease

An infectious disease.

Compare: contagious

infective *adj.* causing infection

An infective organism.

infer *vt.* to conclude from evidence

To infer something from evidence.

A is inferred from B = B implies A.

inference *n.* a conclusion based on evidence

To draw inferences from clinical evidence.

inferential *adj.* relating to inference

A diagnosis of ischaemic heart disease as a result of a positive exercise test is almost always inferential.

inflame *vt.* to cause inflammation
The liver was inflamed by a virus infection.

inflammation *n.* a localized or systemic tissue response to cellular injury characterized by heat, redness, swelling, pain and disordered function
Acute ⟷ chronic inflammation.

inflate *vt.* to distend with gas or fluid
Inflated lungs.
n. inflation

influence *n.* effect
The influence of diet on hormone production.
To /exert/have/ an influence on something.
Compare: effect, impact

influence *vt.* to have an effect on
Physiological factors influence fetal growth.
Compare: affect

influential *adj.* having influence
These genes might be influential in developing disease.

inform *vt.* to tell, give information
They were clearly informed of the risks of driving a car.
Compare: advise

information *n.* knowledge imparted in the form of facts
Information on this phenomenon is beginning to emerge.
Little published information is available on this method.
The questionnaire /sought information on/enquired about/ smoking habits.
There is preliminary information on the detailed structure of HLA antigen molecules.
Ultrasound may provide information about the kidney.
Compare: data, evidence

informative *adj.* supplying information
An informative finding, sign.

informed *adj.* having knowledge
Other family members need informed genetic counselling.
To give one's informed consent.
Compare: consent

infrequent *adj.* rare
Hypokalaemia is an infrequent laboratory finding.

infuse *vt.* to administer an infusion
Acetylcholine was infused into the coronary arteries.

infusion *n.*
1. (continuous) introduction by gravity of a fluid, other than blood, into a vein or other tissue
2. an infused solution

Compare: injection, instillation

ingest *vt.* to take in food or liquid

Two-thirds of ingested lithium from food is absorbed.

Compare: take in

ingestion *n.* intake of food or medications

The chronic ingestion of the drug has caused toxic psychoses.

Compare: intake

ingredient *n.* a component part

The /active ingredient/active agent/active principle/ of a drug.

A multi-ingredient medication.

inherent *adj.* existing as an inseparable part

Compare: intrinsic

inherit *vt.* to receive through genetic transmission

This disorder is inherited.

inhibit *vt.* to slow down or stop a process

Hypophysectomy may inhibit the development of diabetic retinopathy.

adj. inhibitable

Compare: block, prevent, suppress

inhibition *n.* the act, process or result of inhibiting

This activity exerts feedback inhibition on the process.

inhibitor *n.* an inhibiting factor or agent

A coagulation inhibitor.

inhibitory *adj.* relating to inhibition

The drug is inhibitory to RNA = the drug inhibits RNA.

in-hospital *adj.* occurring in hospital

In-hospital respiratory therapy.

initial *adj.* occurring at the beginning

After an initial period of excellent function, rejection occurred.

An initial complaint, finding.

An /initial/starting/ dose.

initiate *vt.* to start

Many aches may be initiated by drugs in common use.

Surgery initiated lymphatic leakage.

n. initiation (of treatment)

inject *vt.* to administer a liquid forcibly into a tissue (by a hypodermic syringe)

The animals were injected with methylcellulose.

The drug was injected intradermally into several sites.

n. injection

injure *vt.* to hurt

He was injured in a road accident.

injurious *adj.* inflicting injury

Injurious to health.

Compare: deleterious, harmful

injury *n.* physical damage

He had sustained multiple injuries.

Injury to a bone from kicks.

Compare: damage

innate *adj.* inborn, congenital

innocent *adj.* harmless

An innocent ⟷ pathological heart murmur.

innocuous *adj.* harmless

Ultrasound examinations are innocuous ⟷ traumatic.

innoxious *adj.* harmless

inoculate *vt.*

1. to introduce microorganisms into a culture medium

To inoculate a specimen onto a transport medium.

2. vaccinate against a disease with active microorganisms

To inoculate a person against yellow fever.

inordinately *adv.* excessively

They were inordinately sensitive to methacholine.

Compare: inappropriately

inpatient *n.* a person admitted to hospital who occupies an adult or child hospital bed for observation, care, diagnosis or treatment (WHO 1)

Opposite: outpatient

inquiry *n.* a systematic investigation

Careful inquiry into the dietary habits of these patients is essential.

insensible *adj.* too small to be perceptible to the senses

/Insensible/imperceptible/ water loss through skin and lungs.

insensitive *adj.*

1. not responsive or susceptible

The tumour was insensitive to chemotherapy.

Compare: resistant

2. lacking physical sensation

Insensitive to pain.

n. insensitivity (to)

insert *n.* something inserted

A vaginal insert, a (drug) package insert.

insert *vt.* to place inside

To insert a catheter, pacemaker, valve prosthesis.

To insert something through something into something.

Compare: implant, introduce

insidious *adj.* developing slowly without being obvious to the patient

The disease is insidious in onset.

The onset of pernicious anaemia is usually insidious.

Compare: indolent

insight *n*. (the result of) understanding

Major insights into the pathogenesis of this disease have been gained in recent years.

The patient had insight into her disease.

These findings provide insights into this phenomenon.

insoluble *adj*. not soluble

Insoluble collagen.

inspissated *adj*. thickened

The bronchioles were filled with inspissated mucus.

n. inspissation

in spite of *prep*. despite, notwithstanding

instance *n*. a case

In this instance, the patient was advised to report immediately to her general practitioner.

instant *adj*. immediate, direct

The drug produced instant relief.

instead of *prep*. in place of

We used drug A instead of drug B.

instil (BE), **instill** (AE) *vt*. to pour or inject drop by drop

A drop of the drug was instilled into the infected eye.

n. instillation; instilment/instillment

institute *vt*. to organize, establish

To institute a study, therapeutic measures.

institutional *adj*. relating to an institution

Institutional care = care in hospital or other appropriate institution.

Institutional mortality.

n. institution

instruct *vt*. to give information

Nurses may instruct patients on their medications.

Compare: educate

instruction *n*. information

Manufacturer's instructions should be followed.

insufficiency *n*. inability to cope with demand

Cardiac insufficiency = heart failure.

Pulmonary insufficiency = more severe lung dysfunction.

Compare: failure

insult *n*. injury, trauma

Repeated ischaemic insults to the myocardium may lead to congestive heart failure.

intact *adj*.

1. untouched

Splenectomized patients ⟷ those with intact spleen.

The antrum was intact in patients who had undergone vagotomy.

intake *n.* what is taken in

Energy intake ⟷ energy expenditure.

High ⟷ low dietary intake of potassium.

Inadequate, poor dietary intake of vitamin D ⟷ excessive intake.

Oral intake of contrast medium.

Strictly controlled, restricted caloric intake.

Compare: ingestion

v. take in

integrate *vi. vt.* to unite with

The virus /integrates/is integrated/ into its host cells.

Compare: incorporate

n. integration

integrity *n.* an unimpaired condition

The destruction of the structural integrity of an organ.

This treatment supports the functional integrity of the systemic circulation.

interact *vi.* to have an effect on each other

Drugs may interact on each other.

interaction *n.* mutual or reciprocal action or influence

Interaction between two drugs may appear as antagonism, additive effects or synergism.

The normal mother–child interaction.

interassay *adj.* occurring between assays

Interassay variations.

intercurrent *adj.* occurring in the middle of a process (e.g. an infection)

An intercurrent infection.

interest *n.* a readiness to be concerned or curious

To have, show, take an interest in a case.

Increasing interest is taken in the possible role of viruses in the aetiology of juvenile-onset diabetes.

To stimulate interest in a phenomenon.

His myxoedema was characterized by a general loss of interest.

The study of this phenomenon has opened a wide area of intensive interest.

interested *adj.* showing or having interest

To be interested in.

interesting *adj.* arousing interest

An interesting finding.

Compare: a superimposed infection

interfere *vi.* to alter, block, slow down, stop, mask or obscure a process

To interfere with a process.

Ascorbic acid may interfere with certain laboratory tests.

interference *n.* the act or process of interfering

Interference with the hepatic blood supply is common in cirrhosis.

This method avoids interference from iodine-containing drugs.

intergroup *adj.* occurring between groups

Intergroup matching.

interindividual *adj.* occurring between or among individual subjects

The drug was bound to plasma proteins with little inter-individual variation.

Compare: between-patient, interpatient, intersubject

intermediate-acting *adj.* with an action of intermediate duration

An intermediate-acting drug.

Compare: long-acting, short-acting

intermittent *adj.* occurring at intervals

Intermittent fever = fever with temperature falling to normal or below normal each day, then rising again.

intermittently *adv.* at intervals

To take a drug intermittently (= not regularly).

interobserver *adj.* occurring between observers

Interobserver disagreement.

interpatient *adj.* between or among patients

Interpatient differences.

interposed *adj.* placed between

The treatment period was two months with an interposed 15-day placebo period between the first and second month.

interpret *vt.* to explain the meaning of

To interpret test results.

These results were interpreted to suggest that . . .

adj. interpretable

n. interpretation

interrupt *vt.* to cause a breach in continuity

The treatment had to be interrupted because of side-effects.

interruption *n.* a breach of continuity

The pain may be relieved by surgical interruption of afferent sensory pathways.

intersperse *vt.* to interrupt with

The wheezing was interspersed with asymptomatic intervals.

intersubject *adj.* between or among subjects

Intersubject variation.

Compare: interindividual, interpatient

interval *n.* a period between two events

The dose was increased by 125 mg at monthly intervals.

intervene *vi.*

1. to occur between points of time

Large meals intervened between long periods of fasting.

2. to take decisive steps in treatment

We were able to intervene therapeutically and to reduce morbidity.

intervention *n.* the act or process of intervening

The intracranial pressure was reduced by operative, surgical intervention.

The symptoms required medical intervention.

intimate *adj.* close in relationship

Magnesium is related to calcium metabolism in an intimate fashion.

intolerant *adj.* unable to tolerate

Patients intolerant of sulphasalazine.

n. intolerance

intractable *adj.* resistant to relief or cure

Certain cases of diabetes are intractable to oral drugs.

Compare: insensitive, recalcitrant, refractory, resistant

intriguing *adj.* interesting

An intriguing postulation.

It is intriguing to speculate whether this mechanism is possible in man.

intrinsic *adj.* belonging to the essential nature of

This defect is intrinsic to the B cell.

Intrinsic asthma = asthma not due to allergic factors.

introduce *vt.*

1. to bring in, present

The drug was introduced in this country in 1970.

Compare: launch, /launch/put/ on to the market

2. to put into

The catheter was introduced through the femoral vein.

Compare: insert

introduction *n.* the act, process or result of introducing

The recent introduction of hepatitis B virus vaccines has opened new approaches for protection.

introductory *adj.* serving to introduce

The introductory chapter of a book.

invade *vt.* to enter a tissue and spread out

Carcinoma invades a tissue.

n. invasion

Compare: encroach

invader *n.* something that invades (a tissue)

A metastatic invader.

invalidate *vt.* to make (test results, etc.) less reliable

Examination of the urine for bacteria can easily be invalidated if insufficient care is taken when the specimen is collected.

invariably *adv.* without a change; always

Acute cholecystitis is usually, but not invariably, associated with gall stones.

invasive *adj.* relating to invasion (into tissues)

Frankly invasive cervical cancer.

Invasive ⟷ non-invasive techniques.

n. invasiveness

investigate *vt.* to examine, study

We investigated these patients for vitamin deficiencies.

investigation *n.* a careful search or examination; study

To carry out/conduct/make/undertake/ an investigation /of/ into/ a disease, in a patient.

A laboratory investigation = a laboratory test.

Our extensive investigation for an aetiological agent was unrewarding.

These drugs are under investigation.

investigational *adj.* relating to investigation

An investigational drug = a drug that is under investigation.

Compare: experimental

investigative *adj.* relating to investigation

An investigative method.

investigator *n.* a researcher

invoke *vt.* to suggest as a cause of a disease

A humoral aetiology of hypercalcaemia of malignancy has usually been invoked only when evidence of skeletal metastasis is lacking.

Compare: implicate, incriminate

involute *vi.* to return to a former condition

The skin lesion may involute spontaneously.

Compare: clear

involution *n.* the act or an instance of involuting

Corticosteroids may hasten the involution of dermatosis.

involve *vt.*

1. to affect

The disease involves arteries.

The eyelids may be involved by angioedema.

2. to be involved /in/with/ a process = to participate in a process
Thrombokinase is involved in the coagulation of blood.
Compare: be concerned in
involvement *n*. the process or result of involving
The involvement of the liver with tuberculosis.
There were 10 cancer patients with abdominal involvement.
These cells /have no direct involvement/are not directly involved/ in the mechanism of hypertension.
irradiate *vt*. to subject to radiation
To irradiate an organ.
Lightly ⟷ heavily irradiated sites.
irradiation *n*.
1. therapeutic or diagnostic use of ionizing radiation
Irradiation treatment by x-rays = radiotherapy.
Irradiation was /delivered/given/ for the relief of neoplastic spinal-cord compression.
She received 6500 cGy of cobalt irradiation to the breast region.
Therapeutic irradiation.
Compare: radiotherapy
2. emission of radiant energy
The underground workers were exposed to solar irradiation between shifts.
Compare: radiation
irreparable *adj*. that cannot be impaired
The irreparable damage associated with arterial thrombosis.
irretrievable *adj*. irreversible
Irretrievable loss of bladder function.
irreversible *adj*. that cannot be brought to a previous condition
Irreversible pulmonary changes.
irrigate *vt*. to flush a wound or a cavity in order to medicate it or to remove a foreign body
To irrigate a wound.
irrigation *n*. the flushing of a wound or a cavity
Neomycin was given by colonic irrigation for intestinal sterilization.
island *n*. an isolated part or area
Islands of active hyperplasia in the thyroid gland.
isolate *vt*.
1. to separate from others for examination in a pure form
To isolate a virus from an organ, /from/in/ a patient.
2. to separate from other persons
To isolate a person suspected of having a disease.

isolated *adj.* occurring alone

This was an isolated finding with otherwise normal renal function.

isolation *n.*

1. separation for examination in pure form from a tissue

The isolation of a virus from a biopsy specimen.

2. social separation of a person who has or is suspected of having a disease

An isolation hospital, ward.

In strict isolation.

Compare: quarantine = a period of isolation, usually consisting of the longest known incubation period of the suspected disease

issue *n.* a point of debate

The issue of whether intrinsic cortical cells degenerate in Alzheimer's disease is unresolved.

To be at issue = to be under consideration.

Compare: problem, question

J

jeopardize, jeopardise *vt.* to risk
  To jeopardize one's health.
  Compare: hazard; risk
judge *vt.* to evaluate
  Biochemical remission was judged by normal 24-hour urinary
  free cortisol concentrations.
  Compare: assess, evaluate
judg(e)ment *n.*
  1. decision, estimate
  To make a judgement.
  2. the capacity for judging correctly
  The occasional removal of a normal appendix does not
  indicate poor surgical judgement.
judicious *adj.* showing good judgement
  The judicious use of rest and drug treatment.
  Opposite: indiscriminate
justify *vt.* to show the correctness of (often used in the passive)
  The use of diazepam to these patients was justified by its
  powerful anxiolytic effects.
  The persistence of these biochemical abnormalities justified
  liver biopsy.
  n. justification

K

keeping *n.* in keeping with = in agreement with
This finding is in keeping with the results of our study.
out of keeping = not in agreement
Compare: in /agreement/concord/ with
keystone *n.* a central principle on which the whole depends
Rifampicin is the keystone of tuberculosis treatment.
Compare: cornerstone, linchpin
kill *vt.* to cause the death of
To kill an experimental animal.
Do not use the euphemism **sacrifice** instead of **kill**.
know *vt.* to be aware of
This syndrome is known to be precipitated by glucocorticoids.
Compare: aware
knowledge *n.* awareness, understanding
/According to current knowledge/on present knowledge/, any
drug-induced liver toxicity is likely to be uncommon.
Detailed knowledge of this phenomenon is still awaited.
The knowledge of this disorder is rapidly deepening, expand-
ing, growing.
To our knowledge such remissions have not been reported.
Compare: awareness, understanding
known *adj.* recognized or diagnosed
Dental care was provided for known hepatitis B carriers.
Timolol should not be used in known asthmatics.
He is a well-known author of many medical textbooks.

L

label *vt.*
1. to describe or classify
Frequently painful and stiff shoulders are labelled as frozen shoulders.
Compare: designate, refer to
2. to make radioactive for tracing = to radiolabel
Kinetic studies with (radio)labelled iron.

laboratory *n.* a room or building used for experiments
Laboratory animals/experimental animals/test animals
Laboratory procedures, laboratory tests, experiments
The laboratory results fell outside the normal range.

laborious *adj.* characterized by great effort
The laborious and often ineffective process of empirical drug trials.
Compare: cumbersome, strenuous

labour *n.* the process whereby fetus, membranes and placenta are expelled from the uterus.
Labour was induced at term by artificial rupture of the membranes.
She was admitted in labour.
She /went into/entered/ spontaneous labour at term.

laboured (BE), **labored** (AE) *adj.* done with difficulty
His respiration was laboured because of pulmonary congestion.
Compare: laborious

lack *n.* absence, unavailability
The atrophy of the intestinal mucosa may result from lack of folic acid.
The lack of a serological marker of infection has, until recently, impeded progress in the understanding of hepatitis.
The underlying defect appears to be a lack of hormone activity. A lack of ⟷ an excess of
Compare: deficiency, deficit

lack *vt.* to be deficient in, to be without
She lacked evidence of this syndrome.

lagging *adj.* developing slowly
The child showed lagging motor development.
Compare: retarded
n. lag

lancinating *adj.* acute, shooting (of pain)

Lancinating pain.

landmark *n.* an anatomical structure used as a point of reference in the study of another structure

This tissue serves as a landmark for somatometric measurements.

lapse *n.* an interval or interruption of time

The time lapse between the injury and the onset of symptoms

Compare: *v.* elapse

largely *adv.* to a large extent

The site of absorption of these drugs in the gut is largely unknown.

late *adj.* occurring late in the course of a disease

Late (-onset) ⟷ early complications after an operation.

Sunken eyes are late signs of dehydration.

latent *adj.* inactive

A latent infection.

Compare: covert, inactive, quiescent, silent

layer *n.* a spreading of some material in a structure

The layers of the aortic wall.

lead *vt.* to cause

These alterations led to hypoxia.

These findings led us to continue our investigations.

Compare: cause, induce, produce, result in

left *adj.* opposite of right

A left hilar mass = a mass of the left hilum.

leg *n.* a part or stage of a study

The three study legs were separated by one week.

Compare: arm

legend *n.* the words that are placed on or under a table or a figure to explain it.

Legends for illustrations should be typed on a separate sheet.

lesion *n.* a pathological or traumatic disorder of the structure or function of a part of the body (such as a wound, abscess, fissure, or tumour)

A benign neoplastic lesion.

A cancer lesion.

A lesion in the upper gastrointestinal tract, such as pyloric stenosis.

A mitotic lesion = a euphemism for **cancer**.

less *adj. comp.* a smaller quantity of

Less oxygen.

Compare: fewer + plural noun

lessen *vi. vt.* to (cause to) become less in size or degree

The pain lessened with rest.

Compare: abate, decrease, diminish

lethal *adj.* causing death

These endotoxins are lethal to adjacent host cells.

level *n.*

1. amount, size or number

The level of consciousness, pain.

2. the ratio of the magnitude of a quantity to a reference value

Blood iron /levels/concentrations.

Compare: content

liability *n.* susceptibility

One characteristic effect of myocardial hypoxia is liability to sudden death.

liable *adj.* susceptible

Obese patients are liable to wound infection.

Compare: apt, disposed, prone, subject, susceptible

liberation *n.* release from the state of combination

Calcintonin is secreted in response to the liberation of pancreatic glucagon.

v. liberate = release

life *n.* opposite of death

Hypercalcaemia may occur during the first few weeks of life.

Their quality of life was excellent after heart transplantation.

There is no satisfactory way of diagnosing this disease in life (= in living subjects).

These attacks interfere with the patient's social and educational life.

This disease may persist for life.

in middle life = in the middle years

life expectancy, life expectation *n.* the number of years an individual can expect to live; expectation of life

Life expectancy is considerably reduced for men and women who suffer a myocardial infarction.

life-saving *adj.* designed for saving life

In severe and prolonged asthma oxygen inhalation often is life-saving.

life situation *n.* circumstances of life

Control of stressful life situations often helps in chronic urticaria.

life-sustaining *adj.* aimed at sustaining life

Life-sustaining treatment such as cardiopulmonary resuscitation.

life-threatening *adj.* threatening to life

Life-threatening infections

lifelong *adj.* lasting through life

Life-long immunity.

The treatment of this disease is life-long.

likelihood *n.* probability

We attempted to reduce the likelihood of recurrences.

limb *n.* arm or leg

Hind/fore limbs = plainly: hind/fore legs; upper limbs = arms, lower limbs = legs.

limit *vt.* to restrict the scope, time, speed, capacity etc.

This discussion is limited to atherosclerosis.

To /limit/to set a limit on/ possibilities.

Compare: confine, restrict

n. limitation

linchpin *n.* an essential element

Drugs remain the linchpin of treatment for Parkinson's disease.

Compare: keystone, mainstay

line *n.* in line with = in agreement with

This suggestion is in line with the findings of other studies.

Compare: agreement, keeping

link *n.* association

The (causal) link between cancer and cigarette smoking.

This disease has a genetic link of susceptibility to carcinogenesis with other age-associated diseases.

link *vt.* to associate, connect

He linked his headache to certain articles of diet.

Many studies have linked smoking /to/with/ earlier natural menopause.

linkage *n.*

1. association

A possible linkage between HLA antigens and alcohol-induced cirrhosis.

2. the association of two genes at different loci on the same chromosome

literature *n.* the body writings in a special field

This has been reported in the literature = Other workers have reported on this.

The literature on specific drugs should be consulted for adverse reactions.

To consult, review, search the literature.

A literature search.

little *adv.* only a small amount (of)

There has been little work on this phenomenon.

The treatment has little or no effect.

load *n.* the quantifiable demand on the functional resources of an organ or organism
The work load of the heart.
Compare: burden, strain
load *vt.* to fill
A syringe loaded with adrenalin
local *adj.* relating to a particular site
Local anaesthesia, medication.
Opposite: general
Note: locoregional = local + regional
localization, localisation *n.* finding the position of
The ultrasound localization of a lesion.
Compare: location
localize, localise *vt.*
1. to determine the place of = to locate
To localize a tumour.
2. to restrict to a certain area
Pain localized to a tooth.
Poorly ⟷ well localized.
locate *vt.*
1. to situate or place
The human insulin gene is located on the short arm of chromosome 11.
2. to determine the place of = to localize
To locate a tumour.
location *n.*
1. the act or action of locating
The location of micrometastases is difficult.
2. a site or position
These glands may be found in unusual locations.
locus *n.* (*pl.* **loci**)
1. a site
The absorptive locus of a drug.
The locus and extent of pulmonary injury.
2. the position of a gene or an allele in a chromosome
long-acting *adj.* with prolonged action
A long-acting drug.
Compare: intermediate-acting, medium-acting, short-acting
long-continued *adj.* continued over a long time
Long-continued/often: long-term/ dextrose infusions.
Long-continued/often: prolonged/ diarrhoea.
Compare: long-standing, long-term, prolonged
longevity *n.* the length of life; a long life
Exercise may extend longevity.

These symptoms usually persist throughout life, but longevity is unaffected.

Compare: life-expectancy

long-held *adj.* held for a long time

A long-held theory.

longitudinal *adj.*

1. relating to the lengthwise dimension

A longitudinal incision of a muscle.

2. relating to a study of a subject or a population over a long period

A longitudinal study.

Opposite: cross-sectional

longitudinally *adv.* in a longitudinal fashion

Human ageing should be studied longitudinally by following the changes occurring in individuals as they grow older.

long-standing *adj.* of long duration

Long-standing rheumatoid arthritis, diarrhoea.

They had a history of long-standing parkinsonian symptoms.

long-term *adj.* occurring over a long period

Chronic or long-term dialysis.

Compare: medium-term, short-term

long term *adv.* for a long time

The patients were in hospital long term.

long term *n.* a long period

In the long term the symptoms subsided.

Recurrences occurred over the long term.

lose *vt.* to suffer deprivation of

He lost consciousness.

losing *adj.* causing the loss of, wasting

Potassium-losing diuretics ⟷ potassium-saving diuretics.

loss *n.* the act or fact of losing

Electrolyte loss ⟷ gain.

Hearing loss = hearing handicap.

Protein loss into the gut.

His tachycardia resulted in loss of consciousness.

There is an abnormally high rate of /fetal loss/fetal deaths/ in pregnant diabetic women.

lost *adj.* no longer available

Days lost from work because of illness.

He was lost to follow-up.

low *adj.* of lesser degree, size or amount than average

The diet was low in residue = it was a low-residue diet.

lower *vi. vt.* to (cause to) decrease

The dose of carbamazepine was lowered.

Compare: decrease, reduce

low-grade *adj.* of small amount

Low-grade fever.

lucid *adj.* relating to a period of sanity or freedom from symptoms

A lucid interval = a disturbance-free period in psychosis or the period between concussion and extradural haemorrhage.

M

magnitude *n.* relative size or extent, importance

The magnitude of an effect, the immune response.

mainstay *n.* the chief support

Since 1879 nitroglycerine has been the mainstay of treatment for angina pectoris.

Compare: cornerstone, keystone, linchpin

maintain *vt.* to keep in an existing state

Most patients can be maintained on this dosage.

Compare: maintenance treatment

They were maintained on mechanical ventilation.

To maintain fluid and electrolyte balance.

Compare: support, sustain

maintenance *n.* upkeep of the existing state

Maintenance treatment = drug treatment with doses that maintain the patient's existing condition.

major *adj.* greater in number, size, importance or significance

A cystic hygroma usually represents a major disruption in the lymphatic system of a fetus.

Alpha-fetoprotein is a major serum protein of early fetal life.

The major blood vessels.

Opposite: minor

majority *n.* most

A specific diagnosis was made in /the majority/most/of these patients.

Opposite: minority

make *vt.* to cause to happen

To make an adjustment, an advance, an analysis, an assessment, an attempt, a comparison, a count, a diagnosis, a determination, an examination, an investigation, a measurement, a modification, an observation, progress, a study of, a survey, a suture.

Compare: carry out, conduct, do

make + comparative adjective = a single synonymous verb

To make better = ameliorate, improve.

To make easier = facilitate, to make worse = aggravate.

make up *vt.*

1. to compensate for

A vitamin A supplement makes up for a deficiency of the vitamin.

2. to prepare a drug

A pharmacy /makes up/dispenses/ prescriptions.

make-up *n.* mental or physical constitution, composition

The biochemical make-up of a cell.

The genetic, emotional make-up of a person.

mal- *combining form* bad(ly)

maldevelopment *n.* defective or abnormal development

The maldevelopment of an organ.

male *adj.* of a male person or animal

It has been suggested that **male** should not be used alone to refer to a man patient or subject.

It can be used as an adjective: a male patient

It can be used collectively: males = boys and men

Compare: female

n. male

malformed *adj.* defectively or abnormally formed

A malformed fetus.

n. malformation

malignant *adj.*

1. life-threatening

Malignant hypertension, malaria.

2. tending to invade, metastasize and terminate in death

A malignant ⟷ benign tumour.

malpractice *n.* neglect of professional duties

A malpractice claim, dispute, suit.

maltreatment *n.* negligent treatment

The doctor was accused of maltreatment.

man *n.* human; human beings as a species

Studies in man and animals.

manage *vt.* to undertake care of

They were managed by chest physicians.

Compare: treat

manageable *adj.* able to be controlled

Obesity should be considered an incurable but manageable disease.

Compare: curable, treatable

management *n.* a programme of medical care

The primary management of the severe pain in many patients with low back pain is the responsibility of the general practitioner.

Compare: a course of therapy; treatment

mandatory *adj.* absolutely necessary

Careful monitoring of these patients is mandatory.

Compare: imperative

manifest *adj.* clinically apparent

Manifest tetany in infantile rickets must be differentiated from convulsions due to other causes.

Compare: clinical, frank, overt

manifest *vt.* to show

Electrolyte depletion may manifest itself by anorexia.

He manifested sensitivity to the drug.

The disease is manifested /as/by/ mental disturbances.

Compare: show

manifestation *n.* sign or symptom

The prevention, arrest, or lessening of neurological manifestations.

manipulation *n.* manual examination or treatment

Manipulation of the calves may dislodge a thrombus.

v. manipulate

manoeuvre (BE), **maneuver** (AE) *n.* a procedure

The planning of /therapeutic manoeuvres/therapy/

manufacture *vt.* to produce

The liver manufactures coagulation factors.

Compare: elaborate, produce

map *vt.* to make a survey of

His visual fields were mapped.

mark *vt.* to characterize

The onset of an attack was marked by severe localized pain.

marked *adj.* clear, noticeable

A marked rise of blood pressure.

Compare: appreciable, clear, distinct, prominent

marker *n.* something used to identify, a mark

Antibody to hepatitis B surface antigen has been used as a marker of previous exposure to hepatitis B virus.

Pancreatic polypeptide is often secreted by pancreatic endocrine tumours and is considered a marker for such tumours.

Compare: hallmark, index, indicator

mask *vt.* to disguise, hide

His mild hyperparathyroidism was not masked by dehydration.

masquerade *vt.* to be disguised

Psittacosis may masquerade as rheumatic fever.

mass *n.* a compact body of matter

A mass such as a metastatic tumour.

Firm, movable, non-tender, palpable abdominal masses were detected.

massive *adj.* considerable; severe

A /massive/high/ dose.

Massive acute myocardial infarction.

Massive/severe/ gastrointestinal haemorrhage.

massively *adj.* highly

Massively/grossly/ obese patients

match *vi. vt.*

1. *vi.* to be equivalent to

Drug A matches drug B in potency.

2. *vt.* to make equivalent to (subjects of a study)

The controls were individually, closely matched with patients for sex, age and residential area.

matched *adj.* corresponding, equal, having similar characteristics

The groups were closely, well matched /for/by/ social class.

matching *adj.* equivalent

Matching blood groups.

Compare: compatible

matching *n.* selection of objects or subjects with similar or identical properties

Donor-recipient matching.

maturation *n.* the state or quality of being mature

To obtain full sexual maturation.

mature *adj.* fully developed

Mature neonates ⟷ /premature/preterm/ infants.

mature *vi.* to become fully developed

maximal *adj.* the greatest possible

The maximal recommended daily dose.

Synonym and *n.*: maximum

meal *n.* a portion of food taken a certain time.

A drug may be taken before meals, at meal time, with meals, after meals, or without regard to meals.

mean *n.* an average

The mean IQ of the study group.

meaning *n.* implications

The meaning of these findings is still unclear.

meaningful *adj.* significant

The numbers of patients were too small for a meaningful analysis.

Note: Sadly, **meaningful** is sometimes a meaningless word.

means *n.* a method of doing

The diagnosis had been made by several means.

by means of = by (using), using

measure *n.*

1. action, procedure

Laser photoradiation is no magic remedy, but almost exclusively a palliative measure of limited value.

2. something used for measuring

The daily sputum volume was used as a measure of response to treatment.

measure *vi. vt.*

    1. *vt.* to determine quantity or degree

    The heart rate was measured from the electrocardiograph.

    2. *vi.* to have a specified extent, amount, etc.

    The tumour measured 10 cm in diameter.

measurement *n.*

    1. the act or process of measuring

    The measurement of bilirubin in amniotic fluid.

    2. amount or degree (usually in the plural)

    The measurements of submaximal bicarbonate output were sensitive indices of abnormal pancreatic function.

mechanically *adv.* by machinery

    Mechanically assisted ventilation.

mechanism *n.* a (physical or chemical) process

    Malnutrition is one mechanism underlying these abnormalities.

    The mechanism by which hormones might stimulate the development of a breast cancer.

    The exact mechanism /for/of/ this phenomenon is not clear.

    The /mechanism/mode/ of action of a drug.

mechanistic *adj.* relating to a mechanism

    This phenomenon has no mechanistic importance.

medical *adj.*

    1. relating to medicine

    A medical examination, problem, student.

    2. of the treatment of a disease by non-surgical means

    Medical ⟷ surgical treatment, medical ⟷ surgical ward.

medication *n.*

    1. administration of drugs

    The patient was discharged on medication.

    2. a drug

    The drug is an effective medication /against/for/ vascular headache.

    He was under medication.

medicine *n.*

    1. the art and science of healing disease

    A student of medicine = a medical student.

    2. treatment of a disease by means other than surgery

    A doctor of medicine.

    The Department of Medicine ⟷ The Department of Surgery.

medium (*pl.* **media/mediums**) *n.* a surrounding substance

A growth medium for bacteria.

The growth of bacteria on a medium.

menopause *n.* the final cessation of menstruation

After the menopause.

adj. menopausal

merit *n.* a positive quality

The merits and limitations of a method.

metabolize, metabolise *vt.* to produce or transform by metabolism

Carbamazepine is metabolized principally to its epoxide.

metabolism *n.*

1. the sum of the processes by which living substance is produced and maintained

2. the sum of the processes by which a substance is processed in the organism

The metabolism of a drug.

adj. metabolic

Compare: fate

metastasis *n.* the (result of) spreading of pathogenic microorganisms or tumour cells from one part of the body to another

Metastasis (=metastatic spread) by the bloodstream.

Metastasis to the fetus is rare.

Metastases (= metastatic growths) were detected in the liver.

metastasize, metastasise *vi.* to transfer by metastasis

Tumours may metastasize to bone.

metastatic *adj.* relating to metastasis

A metastatic growth.

method *n.* the manner of proceeding

Analysis was carried out /by/according to/in accordance with/ the method of Brown *et al*.

microscope *n.* an optical instrument for magnification

Most viruses are invisible in the light microscope.

The cells appeared similar under the scanning electron microscope.

The sample was examined under /a/the/ microscope.

microscopic, microscopical *adj.*

1. using a microscope

Microscopical examination showed a moderate number of neutrophils.

2. too small to be seen except under the microscope

Microscopic particles.

microscopy *n.* examination by use of a microscope

The surface of the cells can be observed, seen /by/on/ scanning electron microscopy

Microscopy showed this.

migrate *vi.* to move from one point to another
    n. migration
migratory *adj.* tending to move
    Migratory arthritis.
mild *adj.* not severe or powerful
    A mild disease, drug, symptom.
    Degrees of severity: mild, moderate, severe
mildly *adv.* in a mild manner.
    His alkaline phosphatase values were mildly raised.
    Compare: slightly
milk *n.* the secretion of the mammary glands
    Human milk
mimic *n.* something that resembles
    General paresis is a great mimic of psychosis.
mimic *vt.* to resemble
    Ischaemic colitis may mimic Crohn's disease.
mimicry *n.* similarity
    One important feature of these tumours is their mimicry of
    malignant neoplasms.
minimal *adj.* small, negligible, smallest possible
    Opposite: maximal
minimize, minimise *vt.*
    1. to reduce to the smallest possible degree
    Pleural fibrosis should be minimized by early treatment.
    Opposite: maximize
    2. to estimate at the lowest possible amount
    A patient may minimize his symptoms.
    Opposite: dramatize
minor *adj.* of smaller number, size, importance or significance
    Minor lymphatic vessels.
    A minor operation.
    Opposite: major
mirror *n.* a thing that reflects something else
    The tongue is often a mirror of disease.
    v. mirror
misapplication *n.* wrong use, misuse
misdiagnose *vt.* to diagnose incorrectly
    The disease was originally misdiagnosed as influenza.
misdiagnosis *n.* incorrect diagnosis
    The initial misdiagnosis resulted from false-positive tests.
misinterpret *vt.* to interpret incorrectly
    The asthma was misinterpreted as pneumonitis.
    Compare: confuse, misdiagnose, mistake for
miss *vt.* to overlook

The occult blood was missed on the first stool examination.

mistake *vt.* to confuse with

In children this disease may be mistaken for febrile convulsions.

misuse *vt.* to use in the wrong way

To misuse drugs.

Compare: abuse

mitigate *vt.* to alleviate

To mitigate the effects of a disease by medical care.

Compare: alleviate, palliate

mix *vt.* to combine or blend ingredients

A fluid can be mixed gently ⟷ vigorously.

mobilization, mobilisation *n.* making ambulant

Early mobilization after operation.

On mobilization she developed sciatic pain.

mobilize, mobilise *vt.* to make ambulant

To mobilize a patient after surgery.

modality *n.* a method

The /treatment/therapeutic/ modalities (=simply: treatment) of accidental hypothermia vary depending on the severity of the condition.

mode *n.* a way or manner of acting

The /mode /mechanism/ of action of this drug is unknown.

The mode of spread of a disease.

model *n.* a representation of something else

Endothelium in culture /is/represents/ a useful model of endothelium *in vivo*.

To construct a model.

moderate *adj.* of middle degree, power or rate

A moderate infection.

Note: degrees of severity: mild, moderate, severe

modify *vt.*

1. to change

To modify a structure.

2. to make milder

To modify the effects of a disease.

n. modification

modulate *vt.* to control

The hypothalamus modulates the activity of the pituitary gland.

Compare: control, govern, regulate

monitor *vt.*

1. to keep under constant surveillance a patient who is under anaesthesia, undergoing operation, etc.

To monitor a patient in the intensive care unit.

2. to examine clinically and by laboratory tests repetitively

To monitor serum iron concentrations.

To monitor side-effects (= to collect, analyse and report upon adverse reactions).

To monitor the growth of a tumour.

Compare: follow, observe

monograph *n.*

1. a book published in a special field

2. a scientific study of a subject

morbid *adj.* diseases, pathological

A morbid condition.

morbidity *n.* the condition of being diseased; the relative incidence of a disease

Attempts to clear blocked cerebral vessels surgically have an unacceptable morbidity.

Compare: frequency, incidence, prevalence

moribund *adj.* in the state of dying

He was admitted moribund.

mortality *n.* death, death rate from a cause

These procedures /carry/are associated with/ a high mortality (rate) = the mortality rate for (patients undergoing) these procedures is high.

mount *vt.*

1. to produce

An individual may sometimes mount an effective immune response against his own tumour.

2. to prepare specimens and slides

To mount slides.

mouth *n.* the oral opening

To give a drug /by mouth/orally.

multi- *combing form* much, many; an abbreviation of **multiple**

multiauthor *adj.* carried out by many cooperative authors

A multiauthor study.

multicentre *adj.* involving many research centres

A multicentre study.

multifactorial *adj.* involving many factors

Multifactorial complications, aetiology.

multiorgan *adj.* involving several body organs

A progressive multiorgan failure.

multiple *adj.* involving more than one at the same time

Multiple-dose vials.

Multiple-drug treatment.

Multiple injuries.

n. multiplicity

multistep *adj.* having many steps

A multistep process.

muted *adj.* silent

In the elderly the signs and symptoms of appendicitis may be muted.

Compare: quiescent, silent

mystifying *adj.* highly unclear

It was mystifying to us why these tumours are invasive despite their small size.

N

native *adj.* normal to a particular location

Native cells ⟷ transfused cells.

Native hormones ⟷ analogues.

Compare: inherent

necessary *adj.* required

Tube feeding is necessary /for/in/ these patients.

necessitate *vt.* to make necessary

Her acute anuric renal failure necessitated haemodialysis.

necropsy *n.* a post-mortem examination

An unexpected observation was made at necropsy.

Compare: autopsy, post-mortem examination

need *n.* requirement

The body's need for calcium, the metabolic need for a hormone.

negative *adj.* indicating absence of a factor

The liver was negative for metastatic carcinoma by liver scan.

The stool examinations were negative for occult blood.

Opposite: positive

neglect *n.* lack of attention

adj. negligent

nervous *adj.*

1. excited, anxious and worried

A nervous patient.

2. of or relating to nerves

A nervous disease, breakdown; the central nervous system.

newborn

1. *adj.* recently born

A newborn baby = a newborn.

2. *n.* a newborn infant, a neonate

When the newborn takes his first breath, he begins to expand his lungs.

non- *prefix*, not

A non-bleeding lesion.

A non-contributory medical history.

A non-excretor of cytomegalovirus.

normal *adj.* in agreement with what is expected, usual or average in a particular statistically defined range

His blood glucose concentration reverted to normal.

His blood pressure was within normal limits.

His diet was normal in fat.

Note: **normal** sometimes occurs as **normo-**: normotensive
v. normalize, normalise
normal *n.* a healthy, undiseased person
Normals and multiple sclerosis patients.
normality *n.* the state of being normal; **normalcy** (AE)
The patient returned to normality after a month in hospital.
notable *adj.* important
Notable clinical features.
Compare: important, prominent
note *vt.*
1. to observe
The investigators noted bacteriuria on the examination.
Compare: find, identify, observe, recognize
2. to record
Any previous shunt procedures were noted.
note *n.* record
In history-taking note was made of exposure to toxins.
A finding of note = an important finding.
notifiable *adj.* denoting disease cases which must be reported to the medical authorities
Salmonellosis is a notifiable disease.
notification *n.* a report of a case of a notifiable disease
Pertussis notifications.
notify *vt.*
1. to report to a medical authority
To notify the health agency of a case of salmonellosis.
2. inform
She notified her physician of lower abdominal pains.
nourishment *n.* food
The patient was unable to take nourishment by mouth.
numbness *n.* a lack of sensation
He presented with numbness of the soles of his feet. The numbness spread up to his knees and was accompanied by weakness of both feet.
nutrient *n.* a nourishing substance
That part of food which nourishes the body consists of both micronutrients and macronutrients.
nutrition *n.* the act or process of nourishing
To ensure adequate nutrition.
Compare: malnutrition
nutritional *adj.* relating to nutrition
Poor nutritional intake.
To maintain a good nutritional state.
The nutrition value of food in carbohydrate.

O

obesity *n.* an excessive amount of bodily fat

Note: **obesity** and **overweight** are not synonyms: obesity refers to an excess of fat, whereas overweight may be due to other variations in body composition apart from excess of fat.

adj. obese

objective *adj.* observable or verifiable by scientific means

Five patients showed symptomatic and objective improvement.

Opposite: subjective

objective *n.* a measurable and attainable state that is expected to exist at a predetermined place and time, as a result of the application of certain procedures and resources (instruments) (WHO 1)

To /accomplish/attain/ the objectives of treatment.

To define, review, update objectives.

obliteration *n.* the act or process of causing to disappear

The obliteration of the insulin response to glucose.

v. obliterate

obscure *adj.* not clear

The exact pathogenesis of this disease is obscure.

obscure *vt.* to make less clear

Corticosteroids may obscure any inflammatory characteristics of this lesion.

observation *n.*

1. the result of observing

Remarkable, valuable observations were made of changes in blood pressure.

2. the state of being observed

Severe symptoms brought the patient under observation.

To keep under close (medical) observation.

observe *vt.*

1. to watch carefully

They should be observed for the possible occurrence of blood dyscrasias.

2. to see, notice

Swelling of the optic disc was seen on ophthalmoscopy.

They had been observed to have cardiac murmurs.

Transient responses may be observed with treatment.

obstacle *n.* something that stands in the way

This disease is frequently an obstacle to the development of the child.

Compare: handicap

obstruct *vt.* to block (up a passage)

An obstructed blood vessel.

n. obstruction

obtain *vt.*

1. to acquire

Specimens were obtained by biopsy.

Urine was obtained by aspiration of the bladder.

2. to achieve

To obtain results by surgical exploration.

To obtain success with a treatment.

obtund *vt.* to make dull

He was obtunded from alcohol, excessive sedation.

obviate *vt.* to make unnecessary

This drug treatment obviates surgery.

Compare: avoid

occult *adj.* hidden, not obvious

An occult spine defect was disclosed by x-ray examination.

Coronary artery disease has a subclinical occult phase.

Occult bleeding, blood.

Opposites: frank, (clinically) manifest, overt

occupational *adj.* of or about an occupation

An occupational disease, hazard.

Occupational health, medicine, therapy.

occur *vi.* to take place

Epigastric discomfort occurred during the first month on the drug.

Restlessness may occur with large doses of the drug.

of *prep.* associated with, related to, relating to

The anaemia of uraemia, the ketosis of starvation.

offender *n.* something that causes injury or disease

Cryptococcus is the most common offender in these fungal infections.

offending *adj.* causing injury or disease

Feathers may be offending agents in asthma.

The offending microorganism = the pathogen.

offset *vt.* to balance

The slight excess of deaths with cancer among control patients was offset by a slight deficit in the deaths without cancer.

Compare: outweigh

offspring *n.* a child or children

The offspring of diabetics tend to be obese.

To produce offspring.

-ology a suffix referring to study of a (branch of a) science

Note: **-ology** is often used to refer to tests or other more concrete things. This usage is condemned by many medical linguists.

Bacteriology (=bacteriological tests) of sputum.

Haematology results = results of haematological studies.

Pathology (sometimes) = disease.

Aetiology = a cause/causes.

on *prep*.

1. referring to place

Pulmonary infiltrates were observed on chest x-ray pictures.

These nurses were working on the intensive care unit.

2. undergoing or subject to treatment with

There was weight loss when the patients were on placebo.

To /place/put/, start, try a patient on digitalis, on postural drainage.

3. during a procedure

Changes were seen on light microscopy.

On admission she had jaundice.

On analysing perinatal mortality in Leeds, we noticed that . . .

On auscultation, section, tomographic scan.

Compare: at autopsy, at laparotomy

4. concerning

An observation on plasma concentrations, a report on cancer.

ongoing *adj*. (mainly AE)

1. in progress

This is an ongoing study and, so far, 20 patients have been admitted.

This study is /ongoing/in progress/.

2. continuous

A vigorous orthopaedic programme which includes ongoing physical therapy.

Ongoing abnormal losses of electrolytes.

Compare: current, continuing, continuous

onset *n*. beginning

The onset of a disease may be insidious, abrupt, explosive and may occur at a certain age.

The onset of blood pressure fall, a menstrual period, treatment.

Chills are common at the onset of bacteraemia.

These attacks may be sudden in onset.

He complained of swelling of rapid onset in the leg.

Diabetes of late onset = late-onset diabetes.

Maturity-onset diabetes; early-onset senile dementia.

open *adj.*

1. not definitely decided

An open question.

2. of a clinical trial: not blind

An open trial ⟷ a blind trial.

operable *adj.* treatable by surgical operation, with a reasonable degree of success

An operable cancer.

Opposite: inoperable

operate *vt.* to do surgery

To operate on a patient, on an organ.

They were operated on for Goldblatt hypertension.

operation *n.* the act or process of operating

To perform an operation on a patient, on an organ.

The diagnosis was confirmed at operation.

operative *adj.* relating to surgery

Operative mortality, results.

operator *n.* a person who operates a machine or an instrument or carries out a medical procedure

Inadequate specimens and serious complications after liver biopsy are the hallmark of an inexperienced operator.

opinion *n.* a view, judgement

Current/prevailing/ opinion is that . . .

Opinions are divided in regard to the merits of this treatment.

opposition *n.* antagonism

This agent acts on carbohydrate metabolism in opposition to insulin.

optimal *adj.* the best

The optimal dosage.

oral *adj.*

1. of, about the mouth

Oral hygiene.

2. given or taken by mouth

Oral drugs = drugs given orally.

Note: **peroral** is rare in English.

Compare: parenteral

order *vt.* to prescribe

A urinanalysis was ordered for these patients.

The doctor ordered surgical treatment.

n. order = prescription

organize, organise *vi. vt.* to form (into) a functioning whole

The cells of a cell culture do not organize into tissue.

orientation *n.* the ability to orient oneself in relation to one's surroundings

oriented *adj.* determined of one's own local and temporal circumstances

He was oriented to person and place.

origin *n.* the primary source

The disease was viral in origin.

originate *vi.* to begin

The bleeding had originated /from/in/ pulmonary capillaries.

Compare: arise

oscillate *vi.* to vary between two values

Blood glucose concentrations oscillate considerably over 24 hours in most insulin-treated diabetics.

Compare: fluctuate, swing

oscillation *n.* a swing

Oscillations in blood glucose concentrations

Compare: fluctuation, swing

other than *prep.* except

Patients who died from diseases other than cancer.

outbreak *n.* sudden occurrence

A large institutional or communal outbreak of a disease.

outcome *n.* result(s)

A favourable outcome was expected in these patients.

The disease has a fatal outcome within a year or two.

The outcome at ages 1 and 3 of children born to diabetic mothers.

Undereducated mothers tend to have poorer pregnancy outcome.

outline *vt.* to show the outlines of

The tumour was outlined by tomography.

outlook *n.* the probable outcome of the individual's disease

The long-term outlook for children with this disease is often poor.

The patient's outlook may be improved by this treatment.

Compare: prognosis

outpatient *n.* a person who makes use of the diagnostic or therapeutic service of a hospital outpatient department but does not occupy a regular hospital bed (WHO 1).

He was discharged from hospital and followed up as an outpatient.

He was observed on an outpatient ambulatory basis.

The implantation was done as an outpatient procedure during a routine clinic visit.

Opposites: hospital patient, inpatient

Compare: a general-practice patient

output *n.* performance

Cardiac output (per minute).

outstanding *adj.* prominent

Headache is the outstanding symptom of brain tumour.

outweigh *vt.* to be more important or weightier than

The risk of death from pulmonary embolism outweighs the risk of serious disability from the consequences of the treatment.

over- prefix; excessive(ly)

An overattended infant; overdiagnosis, overexertion, over-medication, overtreatment.

over *prep.*

1. directly above

There was marked tenderness over the liver.

2. throughout, during a period of time

The drug was given over many months.

Variations in skin thickness over a period.

overall *adj.* general, concerning all parts of a whole

Overall acceleration of clotting was found during the study.

The overall physiological importance of these receptors remains to be determined.

overlap *n.* partial coincidence

The histological overlap of neonatal hepatitis and biliary atresia is considerable.

overlie *vi.* to lie above

Urinary tract stones overlie the bony structure of the sacroiliac region.

Opposite: underlie

overload *n.* an excessive load

Diuretics are needed to eliminate the fluid overload /in/of/ diabetes.

Iron overload may occur in transfusion-dependent patients.

Compare: burden, load

overlook *vt.* to fail to notice

Hypothermia may often be overlooked in minor or major trauma.

Compare: miss

overnight *adj. adv.* lasting the night, for the night

After an overnight fast.

He had to stay in hospital overnight.

overreliance *n.* undue reliance

Diagnostic errors may result from overreliance on laboratory data.

override *vt.* to be more important than

Reduction of left ventricular filling pressure is an urgent necessity which overrides possible metabolic consequences.

Compare: outweigh

overt *adj.* manifest

Overt diabetes mellitus; overt bleeding.

Opposites: occult, quiescent

overview *n.* survey

An overview of observations in laboratory animals.

overweight *adj.* having excessive weight

Overweight people should always be assessed in relation to body build and muscle mass.

overweight *n.* excess weight

Compare: obesity

overwhelming *adj.* overpowering

The overwhelming infection in the urinary fistula was life-threatening.

Compare: generalized

P

pain *n.* the sensation of hurting, suffering

Adjectives of pain: acute, agonizing, boring, burning, crampy, crushing, deep, excruciating, gnawing, intermittent, intense, intractable, lancinating, shooting, stabbing, steady, tearing, throbbing, unremitting

Pain may arise, persist, radiate, recur, resolve, spread, subside.

To /arouse/cause/evoke/give rise to/induce/produce/ pain.

Treatment abolishes, relieves, suppresses pain.

She had pain on swallowing.

She was in pain.

The duration and intensity of pain.

painful *adj.* involving pain

Painful episodes = bouts of pain.

A painful elbow.

palliate *vt.* to relieve (without curing)

To palliate cancer pain, labour pains.

Compare: abate, alleviate, mitigate, relieve

palliation *n.* relief

The object of palliation was to improve the quality of remaining life.

To /achieve/obtain/ palliation of symptoms, of an obstruction.

palliative

1. *adj.* relieving

Palliative management, radiotherapy, treatment.

2. *n.* an alleviating agent

Aspirin is a common palliative for headaches.

palpable *adj.* perceptible by touch

Fetal movements were palpable.

palpate *vt.* to examine by touch and pressure

To palpate the liver.

n. palpation

Note: **palpitate** = (of the heart:) to beat rapidly and strongly

parallel *adj.* corresponding, similar

The synthesis of albumin increased in parallel with the increased loss.

parallel *vt.* to be equal

A marked increase in fungal central nervous system infections has parallelled the decline of tuberculosis.

parameter *n*. a variable whose measure indicates a property that direct methods cannot determine precisely.

The return of a normal diurnal rhythm for cortisol may be an important parameter of cure.

Note: In this broad sense, **parameter** is replaceable with criterion, factor, index, measure, value or variable

parenteral *adj*. introduced otherwise than through the alimentary canal

A parenteral drug, solution.

adv. parenterally

parity *n*. the number of pregnancies that reached or exceeded 28/52 weeks. Stillbirths are included.

Women with a parity of 4.

part *n*. a portion; a role

To take part in a study.

For many years immunology was studied as part of microbiology.

The virus may play an elaborate and less innocuous part in this infection.

participate *vi*. to take part in

He agreed to /participate/take part/ in the trial.

participation *n*. the act of participating

Participation in a study.

Compare: enrolment, inclusion, involvement

particular *adj*. special, specific

It is important to know the particular reasons for the study population being drawn from the general public rather than the hospital outpatient department.

particularly *adv*. especially

The toxicity of aspirin, particularly gastric irritation.

pass *vi. vt*.

1. *vi*. to go through

The drug does not pass the blood–brain barrier.

2. *vt*. to discharge

To pass blood in the urine, stones in the bile.

3. *vt*. to introduce

To pass a catheter into the urinary bladder.

passage *n*.

1. the act of passing

The transplacental passage of an anaesthetic agent.

2. discharge, evacuation

Constipation means difficult or infrequent passage of faeces.

patent *adj*. open, unobstructed

The common bile duct was patent.

n. patency

pathogenic *adj.* causing or able to cause disease

These bacteria are pathogenic to man.

n. pathogenicity

pathognomonic *adj.* characteristic or indicative of a disease

These symptoms, these tests are pathognomonic /for/of/ gout.

Compare: diagnostic, indicative

pathway *n.*

1. a path, course

A lesion in the neural pathways.

The study opened the first pathway into understanding this phenomenon.

2. a chain of reactions in a process

Coagulation pathways.

The metabolic pathways of carbohydrate.

patient *n.* a person receiving medical treatment

A hospital patient.

Compare: inpatient, outpatient

Note: an informal synonym: sufferer

patient population *n.* a specific group of patients as study subjects

This mental hospital admits patients who are referred from hospitals with mixed patient populations.

pattern *n.* the way in which something happens or develops

A hereditary pattern of disease was established.

The dietary patterns of industrialized societies.

We studied the drinking patterns of these patients.

peak *n.* a high value

Peak blood concentrations were reached 30 minutes after oral administration of the drug.

The peaks and troughs in plasma drug concentrations.

Opposites: trough, valley

peak *vi.* to reach a peak

The antibody titres peaked at three months.

penetrate *vi. vt.* to pass into or through something

The knife had penetrated the stomach wall.

Urea penetrates readily into cells.

n. penetration

per cent, percent in or for each hundred

Some 50% of the patients.

percentage *n.* the rate per each hundred

The percentage of symptom-free patients.

percussion *n.* a method of investigating the chest and other parts of the body by tapping, as a diagnostic aid or as a therapeutic method

The outlines of various organs can be roughly plotted by percussion.

perforate *vi. vt.* to make a hole or holes through

The largest diverticulum was perforated.

The ulcer had perforated into the peritoneal cavity.

perforation *n.* the act, action of perforating; the state of being perforated

The perforation of the gut by an ulcer.

perform *vt.* to carry out

To perform an analysis, an autopsy, a biopsy, a determination, an examination, an experiment, an operation, a procedure, a scan, a shunt, a study, surgery, a test.

Perform may seem pompous and is often replaceable by **do**, **make** or **carry out**, if no great accomplishment is being referred to.

performance *n.* the act or process of performing, an accomplishment

Good $\longleftrightarrow$ poor intellectual, mental performance.

period *n.* a portion of time

The accident occurred /at/during/in/ the neonatal period.

periodic *adj.* recurring at (regular) intervals

Periodic examinations.

permanent *adj.* lasting or intended to last without fundamental or marked change

Permanent teeth $\longleftrightarrow$ milk teeth, deciduous teeth.

Permanent visual loss.

permeable *adj.* easy to penetrate

The inflamed synovium is permeable to large molecules.

permit *vt.* to make possible (an action)

Our data do not permit definite conclusions.

Compare: allow

persist *vi.* to continue without interruption, to remain unchanged

A positive Coombs' test may persist for a year.

Patients were encouraged to persist/with/in/ the treatment unless unacceptable side-effects occurred.

persistence, persistency *n.* the act or quality of persisting

The persistence of an antibody, an infecting agent.

persistent *adj.* continuing (without interruption)

Persistent excretion of a virus.

She had a persistent cough.

personally *adj.* directly and not through somebody acting for one

We personally interviewed these patients.

pH *abbr.* potential of hydrogen; used to measure the acidity of or alkalinity of a solution

To maintain the urinary pH at 5.

phase *n.* a distinct period in a development

The disease had entered the anaemic phase.

During/in/ the quiescent, active, acute, chronic phase of the disease.

phenomenon *n.* (*pl.* **phenomena**) an observable occurrence or fact

physician *n.* a doctor of medicine, especially one who treats with drugs

picture *n.* a state or features of

The disease picture.

The histological picture of a disease.

pitfall *n.* a factor that often causes mistakes

A diagnostic pitfall = a source of misdiagnosis.

place *n.*

1. a position, role

There may be a place for empirical permanent pacing in these patients.

This technique may have a useful place in the treatment of cancer.

Compare: role

2. a particular part of space

The catheter was left in place in the trachea.

in place of = instead of

place *vt.*

1. to put in place

A catheter was placed in the cephalic vein.

Catheters were placed in all patients for the administration of fluids.

2. to put on a treatment

They were placed on a therapeutic regimen, on haemodialysis.

placebo *n.* an inactive substance (given instead of a drug)

Administration of placebo.

Placebo tablets = tablets containing inert material.

A placebo-controlled cross-over study.

Placebo-treated patients.

Opposites: active drug, active treatment

placement *n.* positioning

The placement of electrodes for a neurological examination.

plot *vt.* to draw a curve, a diagram

Plasma bilirubin should be measured every five hours and the results plotted on a special chart.

n. plot

pointer *n.* an index

The most useful pointers to hyperthyroidism were loss of weight and restlessness.

Compare: index, marker

policy *n.* a plan of action, approach

To adopt a surgical policy, a treatment policy.

Compare: approach

pool *n.*

1. a group, an aggregation

A bone is a metabolic pool of calcium and phosphate.

These findings suggest the existence of a large pool of drug-resistant organisms in the community.

Compare: reservoir

2. a bank or store

A blood pool.

pool *vt.* to collect (to a pool)

We pooled data from three studies.

pooled *adj.* collected

A single donor or pooled normal adult sera.

poor *adj.* not good

Poor health, results.

population *n.*

1. people in general

Thyroid disorders are more common in these patients than in the general population.

2. a particular group or kind of people

Epidemics occur in military populations.

The study population included patients with vertigo.

portal of entry *n.* the site where an infection enters the body

portend *vt.* to be a sign or warning of, to signify

Multiple organ failure by no means always portends death.

position *n.*

1. a certain arrangement of the body

She assumed the supine position.

She was examined in the sitting position.

2. role

Infections have a less prominent position among causes of prolonged fever now than formerly.

positive *adj.* indicating the existence or presence of that sought or suspected to be present; showing signs of a disease

Strongly positive results were obtained in five patients.

They were positive for the infection.

Opposite: negative

positivity *n.* the quality or state of being positive

Serum parathyroid hormone was not measured owing to positivity to hepatitis B antigen.

possibility *n.* the state or condition of being possible

To examine, explore a possibility.

The important possibilities /of/offered by/ this method.

possible *adj.* capable of occurring

To make possible = to permit, allow.

To make impossible = to prevent.

Compare: conceivable, potential

post- prefix; after

posthospital *adj.* occurring after hospital stay

Posthospital care.

post-mortem examination *n.* the examination of a dead body

Compare: autopsy, necropsy

postoperative *adj.* occurring after operation

Postoperative care, complications.

postoperatively *adv.* after operation

He remained hoarse postoperatively.

postulate *vt.* to propose, suggest

A vascular pathogenesis has been postulated for dermato-myositis.

The cause of the disease is unknown; many causes have been postulated but not confirmed.

n. postulation

Compare: hypothesize, suggest

potency *n.* effect (especially of a drug)

Drug A compares with drug B in analgesic potency.

potent *adj.* important, powerful, effective

Bleeding is a potent factor in increased platelet loss.

This drug is a potent diuretic.

Compare: efficacious, powerful

potential *adj.* possible but not yet actual

Parenteral nutrition has many potential hazards.

potential *n.* latent capacity

A severe handicap might prevent children from achieving their full potential.

potentially *adv.* in a potential manner

A potentially treatable disease.

potentiate *vt.* to make more potent

The drug potentiates the hypotensive effect of antihyper-tensive medications.

powerful *adj.* potent

Vitamin E is a powerful antioxidant.

practice *n.*

1. the usual procedure or method
Radical surgical correction of tetralogy of Fallot has become routine, standard practice.
2. (the place of) the business of a doctor or the number of people using his services
He has a large practice.
Compare: surgery
3. (a doctor's) regular work
The practice of medicine

practise (BE), **practice** (AE) *vt.* to work at a profession
To practise medicine.

pre- *prefix*; before
The prehospital phase of myocardial infarct.
A premalignant condition.
Preterm infants.
Pretransplant findings.
Pretreatment results.

precaution *n.* an action taken to avoid a dangerous event (usually plural)
By /taking/observing/ precautions with all intravenous procedures, the risk of staff acquiring hepatitis B virus will be minimized.
Dietary precautions taken before a test.

precede *vt.* to be earlier than
In epilepsy, focal manifestations precede generalized convulsions.
Compare: announce, herald

precedence *n.* priority
The treatment of this complication takes precedence over all others.

precipitant *n.* a precipitating factor or agent
Depression may act as a precipitant of physical illness.

precipitate *vt.* to cause to occur (abruptly)
His admission was precipitated by respiratory distress.
The slightest pressure precipitated an attack of chest pain.
n. precipitation

precipitous *adj.* abrupt
A precipitous increase in blood pressure.

precise *adj.* exact
We do not know the precise mechanism of this reaction.

preclude *vt.*
1. to prevent, to make impossible
Nausea and vomiting may preclude oral treatment.
2. to rule out

A psychiatric illness does not preclude another painful disease.
The absence of these lesions on pathological examination does
not preclude their existence, as they may be difficult to show
histologically.

predict *vt.* to describe in advance as a result of reasoning
These responses cannot be predicted from previous data.
n. prediction
Compare: foretell

predictive *adj.* serving to predict
The predictive value of a test.
These values were predictive of the clinical course of the disease.

predictor *n.* something that predicts
Serum retinol may be a useful predictor of lung cancer.

predilection *n.* preference
Atherosclerosis has a predilection for coronary, cerebral and
peripheral arteries.
No predilection for age or sex is found in this disease.
Compare: affinity, avidity

predispose *vt.* to make susceptible
The object is often omitted:
Renal impairment strongly predisposes to the accumulation of
toxic levels of the drug.
Alcohol may be a powerful predisposing agent of gout.
Persons genetically predisposed to a disease.

predisposition *n.* state of the body favourable to
A genetic predisposition to a disease.
This gene confers a predisposition to glucose intolerance.

pre-existing *adj.* already existing
Pre-existing/previous/ steroid treatment.

prefer *vt.* to give priority to
Kidney transplantation is preferred /for/in/ most patients with
terminal renal failure.
n. preference

pregnancy *n.* the condition or time of being pregnant, gestation
A full-term uncomplicated pregnancy.
She had had two successful pregnancies.
She was in her third pregnancy.

pregnant *adj.* having unborn offspring in the body
To become pregnant.

preliminary *adj.* preceding something else, as an introduction
A preliminary short report.

premature *adj.* occurring or existing too early
The premature closure of the mitral valve.
Premature /infants/babies/ = those born before term.

premonitory *adj.* giving warning
A premonitory symptom.

preponderance *n.* superiority or excess in number, degree, etc.
The preponderance of men in a study group.

presage *vt.* to give a warning of
The attacks may presage a stroke.
Compare: foretell, herald, precede, predict

prescribe *vt.* to order a treatment
To prescribe a drug for (the treatment of) a disease.
To prescribe a drug (regimen), exercise, rest for a patient.
Compare: order

prescription *n.* a written order from a doctor for a drug
Millions of prescriptions for frusemide are written annually in the UK.
The drug is available on prescription only = It is a prescription drug.

presence *n.* the fact or condition of being present
A lowered plasma cholesterol concentration is found /in/in the presence of/ severe infection.
Opposite: absence

present *adj.*
1. (now) existing
The risk of sepsis is always present with an indwelling catheter.
The symptoms were present or imminent.
Opposite: absent
2. currently available
Present evidence indicates that renal water resorption is passive.
3. this/these
The present study was conducted on 10 patients.
4. at present = now

present
1. *vt.* to introduce for consideration
We present three patients with this disease.
The disease presents several pathophysiological problems.
2. *vi.* to seek medical attention
He presented for medical care.
He presented in the casualty department.
He presented to his local physician, to our hospital with a history of dizziness, to the emergency room.
3. *vi.* to have as its initial sign or symptom
Primary sclerosing cholangitis presents with cholestasis.
The disease may present as acute constipation.
The presenting complaint, symptom.

presentation *n*.
>1. the act of presenting (for medical attention)
>Initial presentation is usually to the general practitioner.
>Patients were studied at presentation for surgery.
>On presentation neurological abnormalities were demonstrable.
>2. the initial signs and/or symptoms
>The disorder had an atypical presentation.

pressure *n*. the force exerted continuously on something
>Blood pressure is the pressure at which the heart pumps blood into the major arteries.
>He had a normal blood pressure.

presume *vt*. to suppose
>We presumed that the patient had complied with our instructions.
>He was treated for presumed meningitis.
>*n*. presumption

presumptive *adj*. based on reasonable belief
>He was admitted with a presumptive diagnosis of pneumonia.
>This patient's presumptive duodenal ulcer has given him little trouble over 20 years.

prevalence *n*. the number of instances of illness or of persons ill, or of any other event such as accidents, in a specified population, without any distinction between new and old cases. The prevalence may be recorded at a stated moment (**point prevalence**) or during a given period of time (**period prevalence**) (WHO 1).
>To reduce the prevalence of a disease in a population.
>*Compare*: incidence

prevalent *adj*. common
>The disease is prevalent in some tropical countries.

prevent *vt*. to keep from occurring
>To prevent accidents, the development of a disease.
>To prevent a disease (from) spreading.
>*adj*. preventable
>*n*. prevention
>*Compare*: forestall, preclude

preventive *adj*. serving to prevent
>Preventive measures, medicine.

previous *adj*. earlier
>Previous/earlier/ studies have shown similar results.
>*Compare*: pre-existing

previously *adv*. earlier
>The analysis was done as previously described.

primary *adj.* first in a series, front-line

Secondary hypercholesterolaemia secondary to diseases, drugs and diets has to be distinguished from primary or familial hypercholesterolaemia.

Metastatic carcinoma with an unknown primary site.

Primary medical care is offered after a patient first presents with symptoms or signs of disease (WHO 1).

prior *adj.* previous

The condition was diagnosed without prior knowledge of the histological results.

prior to *prep.* before

Prior to/plainly: before/ administration of the drug.

problem *n.* a difficulty

To be /confronted/faced/ with problems.

To encounter, identify, meet a problem with a treatment.

To circumvent, correct, eliminate a problem.

To solve a problem = to find an approach, a solution to a problem.

Chromium does not /pose/present/ a nutritional problem.

The same problem applies to all diuretics.

problematic *adj.* difficult to solve or carry out

The treatment of this disease is problematic.

procedure *n.* the practical steps of carrying out a process

To /carry out/undertake/ a procedure.

Diagnostic, laboratory, surgical procedures.

process *n.* a series of events

A metabolic process.

produce *vt.*

1. to bring about, to cause

This disease produces considerable mortality.

This drug produces a marked change in intracranial pressure.

This infection produced liver inflammation.

Compare: bring about, cause, effect, induce

2. to manufacture

Endocrine glands produce hormones.

production *n.* the act, process or result of producing

The production of an atrioventricular block, of hormones.

productive *adj.* producing

A cough productive of brownish sputum.

To be productive of = simply: to produce.

Opposite: non-productive

profound *adj.* deep

Profound hypotension impairs consciousness.

profuse *adj.* abundant

Profuse sweating, discharge.

prognosis *n.* outlook

A careful history is necessary to estimate the patient's prognosis.

The prognosis improves after middle age.

The prognosis is favourable, good ⟷ poor, bleak, grave for this patient, for his intellectual development.

The prognosis with small intestinal tumours depends on the degree of bowel wall involvement.

They had a good prognosis for social independence.

This disease, this patient has a good prognosis.

This sign is associated with a poor prognosis.

Treatment has improved the prognosis for patients with this disease.

Compare: outlook

prognostic *adj.* relating to prognosis

A prognostic factor.

This test has prognostic value.

programme (BE), **program** (AE) *n.* a plan of a course of action

They underwent a programme of investigations.

Compare: battery, panel

progress *n.*

1. the act of progressing

Persistence of these globulin levels may indicate progress to chronicity.

Progress from a clinically undetectable to an advanced stage.

The study was carried out while bleeding was /in progress/ underway.

2. gradual improvement

We have made steady progress in the prevention of childhood accidents.

Compare: advance

progress *vi.* to proceed, to advance

His glomerulonephritis progressed relentlessly to end-stage disease.

His oedema progressed and the drug was discontinued.

progression *n.* the act of progressing

Progression from experimentation with drugs to occasional use.

Steady, swift, stepwise progression to chronic active hepatitis occurred.

The progression of the disease was /arrested/halted/ by treatment.

progressive *adj.* increasing in intensity or severity

The course of the disease was relentlessly progressive.

Progressive disease, loss of weight.

proliferate *vi. vt.* to increase in number

Organisms proliferate in a favourable environment.

To proliferate cells in a medium.

n. proliferation

prolonged *adj.* extended in time

Patients on prolonged drug treatment.

Compare: chronic, long-term, protracted

v. prolong

prolongation *n.* extension in time

The prolongation of survival in adult acute leukaemia.

prominent *adj.*

1. important

Calcification is not a prominent feature of a lung lymphoma.

2. easily seen

This artery was prominent in the x-ray picture.

promise *n.* an indication of good results

This method /holds/offers/shows/ promise for the therapy of several diseases.

promising *adj.* likely to give favourable results

The results of the study were promising.

Compare: encouraging ⟷ disappointing

promote *vt.* to contribute to

Prolonged use of antibiotics may promote the overgrowth of resistant bacteria.

n. promotion

prompt *adj.* performed without delay

Prompt diagnosis and treatment.

prompt *vt.* to move to action

These bronchoscopic findings prompted further investigation.

prone *adj.* disposed to

The ulcer patient may be prone to mental tension.

Addiction-prone individuals.

Compare: apt, liable, subject, susceptible

proneness *n.* the state of being prone

Proneness to periods of depression or elation

Compare: susceptibility

pronounced *adj.* strongly marked

Constipation is usually pronounced in brucellosis.

Compare: marked, prominent

proof *n.* evidence

Conclusive proof is lacking that diminished oestrogen is a factor in arthritis.

Compare: evidence

propagate *vi.* to cause to spread

Popliteal aneurysms may propagate emboli.

n. propagation

Compare: disseminate

propensity *n.* a natural tendency

Malignant melanomas have a variable propensity for invasion and metastasis.

The propensity of leukaemic blast cells towards drug resistance.

This hepatitis has a marked propensity to progress to chronic liver disease.

Compare: avidity, predilection

proponent *n.* one who proposes

The principal proponent of a theory.

Compare: advocate

proportion *n.*

1. the compared relation between two parts; a part of a whole

Asthma attacks due to aspirin-like drugs account for only a small proportion of all deaths from the disease.

Compare: ratio

2. in proportion to = according to, at the rate of ⟷ out of proportion to

In direct proportion to.

The cell membrane surface area was decreased /out of proportion/ /disproportionately/.

The patient's complaints were /out of proportion/disproportionate/ to the findings.

proportional *adj.* being in proportion

Directly ⟷ inversely proportional to

The risk of lung cancer is proportional to daily cigarette consumption.

Opposite: disproportionate

proportionately *adv.* in (correct) proportion

The risk of lung cancer increases proportionately to the number of cigarettes smoked.

Opposite: disproportionately

propose *vt.* to suggest

The author proposed that intestinal metaplasia is associated with gastric cancer.

n. proposition

Compare: postulate, suggest

prospect *n.* a possibility or reasonable hope

One hopeful prospect is that the new developments will make this vaccine more immunogenic.

The operation offered a good prospect for his recovery.

Compare: outlook

prospective *adj.* of a study which is based on future findings, from the research worker's point of view

A prospective follow-up study of this cohort is under way.

Data were recorded in a prospective mode.

Opposite: retrospective

protect *vt.* to keep safe

They should be protected /against/from/ infectious disease.

protection *n.* the act of protecting; the condition of being protected; something that protects

Antibodies /confer/give/offer/ protection against viruses and bacterial pathogens.

protective *adj.* serving to protect

The protective effect of exercise against all-cause mortality.

protocol *n.* the exact instructions for the administration of a test or treatment

A bone marrow transplantation protocol.

A deviation from the study protocol.

protracted *adj.* extended in time

Protracted haemorrhage, mental stress, urinary haemoglobin loss

Compare: long-term, prolonged

prove *vi. vt.*

1. *vt.* to show or establish (*participate* and *adj.* = **proved** or **proven**)

The sedative effects of this drug have been proven.

The treatment of hyperlipidaemia has not been proved to prevent atherosclerosis.

Biopsy-proven Hodgkin's disease, culture-proven cases of a viral disease, x-ray proven conditions.

They had 10 proved sites of ectopic ACTH production.

Opposite: disprove

2. *vi.* to turn out (to be)

Our patient /proved to have/had/ resistant organisms.

Treatment A /proved/was/ less effective than treatment B.

provide *vt.* to supply

The hospital provided excellent exercise facilities for patients.

This finding provides support or evidence for our theory, for our suggestion.

This technique provides an estimate, a measure of myocardial blood flow.

provocation *n*. causation, stimulation

The provocation of an infection, of a response.

provocative *adj*. causing illness

Exposure to provocative agents.

provoke *vt*. to cause

To provoke illness, a reaction.

Compare: bring about, elicit

proximal *adj*. nearest or nearer to the point of reference

A colonic obstruction proximal to the splenic flexure.

Opposite: distal

psychic *adj*. mental

Psychic/mental/ tension.

publication *n*. the act, process or product of publishing

To submit, accept an article for publication.

publish *vt*. to make known generally (usually through a book or a journal)

Many studies have been published on this syndrome.

Published studies support this finding.

Reports of investigations published from various centres

pulse *n*. the rhythmic expansion of an artery produced by heart contractions

The peripheral pulses were bounding, full, irregular, rapid, thready.

The pulse rate.

puncture *n*.

A lumbar puncture yielded clear, colourless cerebrospinal fluid.

v. puncture

purgation *n*. the act or process of purging (of the bowels)

Bowel preparation consisted of thorough purgation before surgery.

v. purge

purulent *adj*. containing pus

A purulent wound.

Purulent discharge.

pus *n*. a thick fluid produced by inflammation

Q

quality *n*. characteristics, nature

The quality and pattern of sleep.

The quality of medical care.

quantity *n*. an amount or a number

In pregnancy, oestrogens are produced in large quantities = Large quantities of oestrogens are produced in pregnancy.

question *n*.

1. a problem

Many questions remain /to be answered/open.

Several questions arise.

These studies, these workers raised several questions.

This is an /open/unanswered/unresolved/ question.

We offer a definitive answer to this question.

2. consideration

The patient in question = the patient under /consideration/ discussion/.

question *vt*.

1. to ask questions

The patients were questioned about the presence of headache.

2. to doubt

The workers questioned the wisdom, use of giving aggressive chemotherapy to these patients.

questionable *adj*. doubtful

The value of this treatment is questionable.

questionnaire *n*. a form with a set of questions

A questionnaire asking about details of infertility was sent to patients.

A questionnaire was administered by telephone.

A questionnaire on the side-effects of the drug.

They completed a /self-administered/self-completion/ questionnaire.

To collect data with a questionnaire.

Inquiry by postal questionnaire.

quiescent *adj*. silent

The symptoms remained quiescent for 10 weeks.

Compare: dormant, inactive, latent, silent

R

radiation *n.* electromagnetic waves; radiation therapy

The radiation dose = the irradiation dose.

Radiation-induced leukaemia.

Radiation treatment/radiotherapy/ by x-rays.

radical *adj.* directed to the root of a disease

Radical surgery.

radiograph *n.* an x-ray picture

Lesions were detected on a chest radiograph/film.

radiograph *adj.* relating to a radiograph

The radiographic abnormalities (shown) in Fig. 1.

The radiographic view in Fig. 1.

The radiographic appearance of the bone.

Radiographic evidence, lesions.

n. a radiogram or a radiograph, also called roentgenogram

radiotherapy *n.* the treatment of a disease by radioactive substances

She received /radiotherapy/irradiation/radiation/ to the tumour site.

raise *vt.* to make higher in amount, degree, size, etc.

Her blood glucose concentrations were slightly raised.

Compare: elevate, increase

randomly *adv.* in a random manner

Patients were randomly /assigned/allocated/, selected /for/to/ a four-week treatment period.

random *adj.* randomized

Random allocation of patients to groups.

They were studied in a random double-blind fashion.

randomize, randomise *vt.* to apply randomization to

A randomized double-blind cross-over /technique/design/.

The treatment sequence, entry to the trial was randomized by Latin squares.

They were randomized into four groups, to receive treatment with the drug.

n. randomization, randomisation

range *n.* the limits of variation

All his joints had a full range of movement.

All patients were in the age range of 15 to 25 years.

The drug is effectively in a wide range of clinical situations.

The serum prolactin concentration /fell/was/ within the normal /range/limits/.

Compare: spectrum

range *vi.* to vary between limits

Their ages ranged from 15 to 25 years.

rare *adj.* uncommon

Complications are rare with this technique.

n. rarity

Compare: infrequent

rate *n.* the quantity, amount, or degree of something measured by its relation to something else

The heart rate, respiratory rate.

The fertility, morbidity, mortality rate.

To infuse glucose at a certain rate.

rate *vt.* to assess

Improvement in individual symptoms was rated on a four-point scale.

Compare: assess, grade

rather than *prep.* by preference

Rather than use these individuals as study subjects, we used healthy hospital staff.

ratio *n.* the relationship between two numbers or quantities

The benefit-to-risk ratio in drug treatment: risks must be weighed against benefits, benefits must outweigh the possible risks.

The ratio of polyunsaturated to saturated fats in the diet.

The sex ratio of mortality rates from coronary heart disease.

This tumour is found in men more often than women by a ratio of 3:1.

rationale *n.* the basic logical principle

The rationale for postoperative radiation is to prevent local or regional relapse of the cancer.

re- *prefix*; again

The readministration of a drug, readmission to hospital.

The reappearance of symptoms, the recurrence of cancer.

Retreatment.

reach *vt.*

1. to get to

An experienced colonoscopist can easily reach the caecum.

2. to attain

The drug reaches high concentrations in blood and tissues.

react *vi.* to respond to

To react to a stimulus.

reaction *n.* an action due to a stimulus

A brisk reaction with a drug.

A reflex reaction to pain.

The adverse reactions to a drug = side-effects.

To provoke an immune reaction.

reactivation *n.* the process or result of becoming active again

The reactivation of a disease.

Compare: flare-up, recurrence, relapse

reactivity *n.* responsiveness

Immunization induces reactivity to antigenic substances.

Strong ⟷ weak reactivity.

adj. reactive

read *vt.* to interpret

To read an electrocardiogram, a skin test.

readily *adv.* easily

The drug is readily absorbed from the gastrointestinal tract.

readiness *n.* the state of being ready or prepared

This equipment is kept in readiness until danger has passed.

real *adj.* genuine, not artificial or false

Real ⟷ simulated therapy.

Compare: true

recalcitrant *adj.* not susceptible to control

The pruritus was recalcitrant to conventional measures.

Compare: intractable, refractory, resistant

receive *vt.*

1. to take or get

To receive a drug, a treatment.

2. to be the subject of

The blood cultures received prolonged incubation.

recidivation *n.* the relapse or recurrence of a disease

recidivation is rare in English. Use **recurrence**.

recipient *n.* one who receives (a transplant)

Opposite: donor

recognition *n.* the act or action of recognizing

Early recognition of pneumococcal pneumonia saves many patients.

recognizable, recognisable *adj.* identifiable

In most cases this disease has no recognizable cause.

recognize, recognise *vt.* to identify, be aware of, know

Rubella was /recognized/identified/ as a specific cause of the abnormality.

The patient may /recognize/notice/ complete A-V nodal block as a slower heart rate.

The association between alcoholism and accidental injury is well /recognized/known/.

Myocarditis is a /recognized/known/ complication of infectious mononucleosis.

recognition *n.* identification

The recognition of a cyst on nephrotomographic examination.

recommend *vt.* to present as a good choice

This dose is recommended for adults.

record *n.*

1. recorded facts

The medical record of a patient = a record of all his illnesses and the treatments he has received.

The obstetric records /on/of/ these women.

They were given a /diary/record book/ and asked to answer each evening a set of questions about various symptoms.

2. performance

Some countries have a poor record in treating renal failure.

record *vt.*

1. to preserve in writing

At each visit weight was recorded.

Clinical details were recorded for all reported cases.

2. to register

His tachycardia was recorded on the electrocardiograph.

recover *vi. vt.*

1. *vt.* to get back, regain

They recovered good neurological function.

2. *vi.* to return to normal health

He recovered from the disease.

Compare: recuperate

3. *vt.* to find

Cytomegalovirus was recovered from urine and saliva.

recovery *n.*

1. return to health

To induce recovery by treatment.

He made a good ⟷ poor /complete/full/recovery; an /uncomplicated/uneventful/uninterrupted/ recovery from the infarction.

2. finding

The recovery of a microorganism from a site.

recrudescence *n.* recurrence of symptoms after temporary abatement (after some days or weeks)

Recrudescence of chest pain.

Compare: recurrence, relapse

recrudescent *adj.* appearing again

Recrudescent symptoms.

recruit *vt.* to obtain subjects for a study

Ten patients were recruited for the study by means of clinical referrals.

Compare: enrol

recruitment *n.* the act of recruiting subjects for a study

Recruitment was by public advertisement.

rectify *vt.* to correct

This deficiency of dopamine was rectified by levodopa.

Compare: correct

recumbent *adj.* lying down

A recumbent hospitalized patient.

They remained recumbent for one hour after injection.

n. recumbency

recuperate *vi.* to get well again

To recuperate from illness.

Compare: recover

recur *vi.* to occur again

The infection recurred six months later.

Compare: return

recurrence *n.* the return of a disease after a remission

He developed a recurrence of the cancer.

Compare: reactivation, recrudescence, relapse

recurrent *adj.* occurring again

Recurrent infections.

reduce *vt.* to make smaller in number, amount, degree, etc.; to decrease

Reduce from something to something, in a continuous process, often by a definite amount.

To reduce pituitary activity, secretion of a hormone, the heart rate.

The verb is often used in the passive:

Blood pressure was sharply reduced in all patients.

reduction *n.* the act or action of reducing, the amount reduced

A 30% reduction in the mortality rate.

re-evaluate *vt.* to examine again

They were re-evaluated periodically to rule out any intercurrent infection.

n. re-evaluation

Compare: review

refer *vt.*

1. to send over for treatment to another practitioner or institution

He was referred to a cardiologist for evaluation of a heart murmur, to us for treatment with the diagnosis of asthma.

Hospital-referred patients = patients referred to hospital.

2. to perceive pain signals as originating from

Inflammation of the liver causes pain to be felt in the shoulder = the pain is referred to the shoulder.

The back pain was interpreted as referred pain from a diseased gall bladder.

3. to speak of

Lymphokines are referred to as the chemical mediators of cellular immunity.

4. to relate to

Pure red blood cell aplasia refers to cases in which only the red cells and their precursors are affected.

referable *adj.* attributable to

The symptoms were referable to the affected visceral structures.

reference *n.*

1. a mention

A reference to other reports published on the same subject.

to make reference to = to refer to

2. **with special reference to** = with special emphasis on

referral *n.*

1. sending a patient for care to another practitioner or institution

Referrals to medical consultants /by/from/ general practitioners.

These signs merit prompt referral to a centre.

A referral centre = a treatment centre to which patients are referred.

2. perception of pain signals as originating from

Referral of symptoms of appendicitis to the left side of the abdomen.

reflux *n.* a flowing back

The reflux of duodenal contents into the stomach.

refractory *adj.* resistant or unresponsive to treatment

Patients refractory to other antihypertensive agents usually remain responsive to diazoxide.

Drug-refractory tachycardia.

Compare: recalcitrant, resistant

refusal *n.* an expression of unwillingness

Refusal of feeds by an infant.

v. refuse

refuse *vt.* to reject

The patient may refuse medical help.

refute *vt.* to deny or show the inaccuracy of

To refute a diagnosis.

Opposites: confirm, support

regain *vt.* to recover

To regain normal renal function, to regain one's appetite.

regimen *n.* a systematic plan of treatment

The drug was given in a prolonged regimen.

regime is rare in this sense.

region *n.* a largish area

He complained of pain in the region of the joint.

regional *adj.* pertaining to a region

Most patients with low back pain have a regional backache –
i.e. one that is not caused by systemic disease.

Regional myocardial contractile dysfunction.

regression *n.* a progressive abatement of symptoms or a disease

Marked regression of xanthomas.

Compare: reversal

regulate *vt.* to control

This hormone regulates fluid and electrolyte homeostasis.

n. regulation

Compare: control, govern, modulate

regulatory *adj.* pertaining to regulation

Cardiovascular regulatory functions.

rehabilitation *n.* restoration of former form and function after
injury or illness

Rehabilitation after myocardial infarction.

v. rehabilitate

reject *vt.* to fail to accept

Non-compliers were /rejected for/excluded from/ the trial.

The body may reject a transplant.

rejection *n.* a case of rejecting

A rejection episode occurred after renal transplant.

Graft rejection occurs if a graft is transplanted in defiance of
the blood group barriers normally present in blood transfusions.

relapse *vi.* to become ill after an apparent cessation of a disease

He had relapsed from previous chemotherapy.

The resuscitated patient may relapse into cardiac arrest.

Relapsing fever = fever in which febrile periods alternate with
one or several days of normal temperature.

Relapsing-remitting sclerosis ⟷ stable sclerosis.

relapse *n.* a recurrence of disease progression after some weeks or
months of abatement

Silent ⟷ symptomatic relapse.

Compare: recrudescence = recurrence after some days or
weeks

relate *vt.*

1. to show or establish a causal relation

The study attempted to relate blood lead concentrations to environmental exposure.

Compare: associate, connect, link

2. to tell

The patient relates his symptoms.

Compare: inform

related *adj.* associated

Brain infarction is intimately related to blood coagulation.

The classical manifestations of anaemia are directly related to its severity.

Sleep-related hypoxaemia.

relation *n.* an association, a connection

Several studies have shown an inverse (⟷ direct) relation between vitamin A intake and cancer.

The severity of this symptom /bears/has/ little relation to disease activity.

Mortality rates were studied in relation to weight and height.

Compare: association, connection, linkage, relationship

relationship *n.* relation

Certain factors may disguise, obscure a relationship.

The relationship between the clinical symptoms of the disease and serum calcium concentrations is often /poor/weak/(⟷ clear).

The relationship of these defects to the development of malignant diseases remains to be confirmed.

Compare: association, correlation

relative *n.* a person related by blood or marriage, family members

First-degree relatives.

The procedures could not be carried out without permission of a relative.

relative to *adj.* connected with, in relation to

A deficit of body water relative to sodium.

The problems /relative/relating/ to this disease.

relative to *adv.* in relation to, in proportion to

A hot nodule has increased uptake relative to the remainder of the gland.

relax *vi. vt.* to (cause to) become less stiff or tense

On expiration the muscle fibres of the diaphragm relax (⟷ contract).

Tranquillizers tend to relax such patients.

release *vt.* to liberate

To release a substance via the blood stream into an organ.

n. release

relevant *adj.* having direct bearing on the subject

He had no relevant medical history apart from recurrent back pain.

These symptoms may be relevant to the development of cancer.

relevance *n.* significance

The relevance of the findings of a study to clinical practice

Compare: application, implication

relief *n.* alleviation of symptoms

A treatment /brings/gives/provides/produces/ relief of symptoms.

The patient /gains/obtains/ relief /by/from/with/ a drug, treatment.

He was given a drug /for relief of/to provide relief from/ itching.

Prompt and prolonged relief.

relieve *vt.* to alleviate, to lessen

The pain was relieved by an analgesic.

Compare: alleviate, assuage, mitigate, palliate

rely on *vi.* to depend on

This method relies on measuring the total concentration of the drug in plasma.

Compare: depend on

remain *vi.* to be left to be done

The clinical applications of these observations remain to be determined.

The implications of these findings /remain/have yet/ to be explored.

remarkable *adj.* noteworthy

The pulmonary lobe was remarkable for its irregular shape.

remediable *adj.* capable of being cured

Surgically remediable anomalies.

Compare: curable, treatable

remedy *n.* a medicine or treatment

The use of this treatment as a remedy for disease is still limited.

v. remedy

reminiscent *adj.* suggestive

The histological picture was reminiscent of hypersensitivity.

Compare: indicative, suggestive of

remission *n.* (the period of) abatement of symptoms

The treatment /achieved/affected/induced/produced//continuous/sustained/ and complete (⟷ partial) remission.

The patient /achieved/attained/entered/reached/ remission, and remained in remission.

The drug maintained the patient in remission.

He was discharged in complete remission.

The spontaneous, permanent remission of a disease in a patient.

Opposite: exacerbation; repeated exacerbations and remissions = fluctuations

Compare: remittance, resolution

remit *vi*. to diminish symptoms, to decrease in intensity

The disease remitted at six months.

The pain remitted completely.

remittent *adj*. fluctuating in intensity

Remittent fever = daily rise and fall of body temperature, without return to normal.

Compare: intermittent

n. remittent

remove *vt*. to take away

The patient was removed from the contaminated environment and his contaminated clothing was removed.

The solvent was removed by suction.

n. removal

render *vt*. to cause to be

Sodium bicarbonate /rendered/plainly: made/ their urine neutral.

repair *n*. restoration of damaged or diseased tissues by the growth of healthy new cells or surgical apposition

Cell, tissue repair.

v. repair

repeat *adj*. something that is done again

A repeat renal angiogram.

Repeat prescriptions.

replace *vt*. to put something in the place of something else

Attempts were made to replace a loss in red blood cell mass by blood transfusion, with transfused cells.

Compare: make up for, substitute

replacement *n*. the act of replacing

Bone marrow replacement by tumour.

Replacement therapy = therapy that replaces deficient formation or loss of body products with the natural body products or synthetic substitutes.

Hormone, fluid replacement therapy.

replenish *vt*. to fill up again

To replenish depleted body iron stores.

n. replenishment

report *vt*.

1. to publish a report
We report (on) a patient who presented with polymyositis.
We report (on) the use of this method in 10 patients.
The drug has been reported as producing side-effects.
They were reported as having epilepsy.
The mortality rate reported for this disease, these patients.
Recovery rates reported from alcoholic clinics.
2. to tell of
They reported complete relief of symptoms.
Compare: inform, relate

report *n.* a published account
Published reports strongly suggest this.
Personal report/communication = simply: conversation, letter, etc.

reportedly *adv.* according to report(s)
The risk of death in these patients is reportedly increased in the presence of ventricular premature beats.

reproductive *adj.* producing offspring
Women of /reproductive/child-bearing/ age.

require *vt.* to need
He required surgery for relief of pain.
The method required careful assessment.

requirement *n.* a need
His amino acid requirement was /met/satisfied/, but not exceeded.
The high requirement of vitamin D (= need for massive doses).
requirement often refers to an /immediate/temporary/transient/ state, while **need** refers to a permanent state.

rescue *vt.* to save
Drug treatment in established cardiac shock may rescue a few patients.

research *vt.* to study
To research a subject = simply: to study a subject.

research *n.* advanced study of a subject
Active research into cell-mediated immunity is in progress.
To /carry out/do/ research.
These findings opened a new field of research /into/on/ inflammatory reactions.
A research team.

research worker *n.* one who carries out research
His report aroused controversy among British research workers.
Often briefly: worker

resect *vt.* to remove (part of) an organ or other structure surgically
A large-bowel polyp was resected.
Compare: dissect, excise

resection *n.* surgical removal
They had undergone surgical resection of lung cancer.

resemble *vt.* to be similar to
A gross excess of this hormone may cause symptoms which superficially resemble psychiatric syndromes.

reserve *n.* a store for future use
Body reserves of fat.

reserve *vt.* to keep or give for a specific purpose
Regional sympathectomy is reserved for patients with progressive disability (relief only for 1–2 years).

reservoir *n.* a (large) supply or store
To eradicate a reservoir of infection by vaccination.
Compare: pool

residual *adj.* remaining
Many survivors of this disease are left with residual deficits.
The manifestations of rheumatic fever subsided without residual effects.

residue *n.* solid material left behind after some process, a remainder
This diet results in large amounts of residue.
A high-residue ⟷ low-residue diet.

resistance *n.*
1. an inherent capacity for resisting
Obesity imposes a demonstrable resistance to the physiological action of insulin.
2. the ability of an organism to remain unaffected by harmful environmental agents
The bacteria acquired drug resistance = the bacteria became drug-resistant.

resistant *adj.* unresponsive to treatment
Five bacterial strains were resistant to the drug.
Resistant supraventricular arrhythmias.
Compare: intractable, recalcitrant, refractory

resolution *n.*
1. subsidence of symptoms
Prompt resolution of the swelling was achieved.
2. breaking up into parts
The resolution of urate deposits.

resolve *vi. vt.*
1. to (cause to) subside
Her pyrexia and tachycardia resolved after 10 days.

2. to break up into parts, to dissolve
To resolve a deposit of urates.

respectively *adv.* each separately in the order given
One patient died of cancer, one of cardiac arrest and one of septicaemia; their ages were 7, 56 and 31, respectively.
Plasma concentrations of amino acids and fatty acids are raised, indicating catabolism of tissue protein and triglyceride, respectively.

respond *vi.* to react
He responded to corticosteroid treatment with a marked increase in intraocular pressure.
He responded poorly to the drug.

responder *n.* one who responds
A responder to a questionnaire, to a treatment.

response *n.* an action due to the application of a stimulus
He mounted an effective immune response against his own tumour.
They/made/showed/a /good/favourable/ ⟷ poor response to treatment.
We /attained/elicited/obtained/produced/provoked/ a good, prompt response with the treatment.
An antigen produces an immune response = an immune response occurs after exposure to antigen.
The onset, intensity and duration of the response.
The total dose was determined by clinical response.
He increased his water intake in response to thirst.

responsible for *adj.* being the cause of
Factor A is responsible for disorder B = Disorder B is due to factor A.
The toxicity of alcohol can be held directly responsible for alcoholic liver disease.

responsive *adj.* reactive
He /was responsive/briefly: responded/ to hormone treatment.
n. responsiveness
Opposite: unresponsive
Other adjectives expressing various aspects of responsiveness to treatment: amenable, (in)curable, recalcitrant, refractory, (ir)reversible, (in)sensitive, (in)tolerant, (un)treatable

rest *n.* inactivity after exertion or work
At rest ⟷ during exercise, on exertion.
He was on bed rest.

resting *adj.* relating to rest
Resting blood pressure level = blood pressure (measured when the subject is) at rest.

restoration *n.* (causing) return to a previous state (of health)
  The restoration of a normal blood pressure.
  Compare: recovery
restore *vt.* to return
  His vision was restored.
  To restore an individual to health from illness.
  Compare: return, reverse
restrain *vt.* to keep within limits
  His diet was restricted to easily digested high-carbohydrate foods.
  We restricted his fluid intake.
restrict *vt.* limit
  Viral replication was restricted to cells that made growth hormone.
restriction *n.* the act of restricting, something that restricts
  Dietary restrictions.
  To impose a fluid restriction.
result *n.* something that occurs as a consequence, issue or conclusion of an action or event
  To derive, obtain results from a study, treatment.
  A study, treatment yields results.
  as a/the result of = often better: because of
  with the result that = so that
result *vi.*
  1. result from = to occur as a consequence of
  Metabolic bone disease may result from vitamin D deficiency.
  Compare: vitamin D deficiency may result in bone disease.
  2. result in = to have as a result
  These investigations resulted in a diagnosis of gastric carcinoma.
  resulting from = due to, caused by
resume *vt.* to start again after a pause
  Oral feeding should not be resumed too early after peritonitis.
  The patient was able to resume her customary physical activities.
resuscitation *n.* bringing back to life or consciousness
  To apply resuscitation.
  v. resuscitate
retain *vt.* to keep in position
  Asbestos fibres are likely to be retained in the alveoli.
  n. retention
retard *vt.* to slow down
  Coagulation is retarded by cold.
  Salicylates retard wound healing.

A mentally retarded person.

n. retardation

Opposites: accelerate, hasten, speed ⟷ slow

retention *n.* abnormal retaining (of a fluid within the body)

Chronic urinary retention due to bladder neck obstruction.

Fluid retention may occur in obese subjects.

retrospect *n.* in retrospect = in surveying medical records or re-evaluating events

In retrospect, all cytomegalovirus cultures for four patients were negative.

retrospective *n.* a retrospective study is a study of data of past events

A retrospective study of data from a registry for fetal surgery.

Opposite: prospective study

retrospectively *adv.* according to a retrospective study design

Avoidable factors can be identified retrospectively in many patients who have died from this disease.

return *vi.*

1. to recur

His ascites returned.

2. to go back to

He returned to gainful employment, normal function, occupational work.

reveal *vt.* to show

X-ray studies /revealed/showed/ multiple fractures.

Compare: disclose, show

reversal *n.* the act or instance of reversing a disease in its course

The treatment depends on the reversal of the underlying disorder or withdrawal of the offending drug.

reverse *vt.* to turn a disease in its course

Exogenous glucose was given to restore normal cellular use and thus reverse the ketoacidosis.

He had reduced visual acuity which was reversed when the drug was stopped.

reversible *adj.* capable of being reversed

This symptom is reversible on withdrawal of the drug.

Opposite: irreversible

revert *vi.* to go back to a former condition

Four patients already in renal failure reverted to normal.

Compare: involute, return

review *vt.*

1. to make a survey

We have reviewed the management of acute cholecystitis in this country between 1975 and 1979.

2. to examine critically, to re-evaluate

The use of drugs should be reviewed with the patient.

To review vaccination policies.

review *n.*

1. a survey

A review of hospital records.

A review of the literature = a literature review.

2. re-evaluation

All ulcerative colitis patients require careful, frequent reviews for evidence of carcinoma.

Liver function was monitored and a review cholecystogram performed at six months.

revise *vt.* to change after reconsideration

Their antibiotic treatment was revised when necessary.

n. revision

rich in *adj.* having a large proportion of

Foods rich in gel-forming fibre.

Compare: high in

rigidly *adj.* strictly

All medication in the group was rigidly supervised.

rise *n.* the act or instance of rising, an increase in amount

A sharp rise in temperature.

Opposites: decrease, drop, fall

Compare: increase

rise *vi.* to become higher, to increase

The temperature rose daily in steps.

Opposites: decrease, drop, fall

Compare: increase

risk *n.* possibility of loss, harm or injury

There are always risks associated with surgery.

These abnormalities put the patients at the risk of liver disease.

These patients /are at risk of/run a risk of/ permanent disablement.

This technique carries some risk of impairing sphincter control, a risk to life.

We must identify, lower this risk in psychiatric patients.

The beneficial effects of the drug are offset by a risk of cardiac arrhythmias.

The risks must be weighed against the possible benefits.

adj. low-risk, moderate-risk, high-risk

Note: *risky* is not used in ME papers.

risk-benefit *adj.* relating to a comparative analysis of possible risks and benefits

The /risk-benefit/risk versus benefit/ ratio of pertussis clearly favours routine immunization.

Compare: a cost-benefit analysis

risk factor *n.* something that presents a risk

Cigarette smoking is a /major/strong/ risk factor for coronary heart disease.

risk; high-risk, high risk ⟷ **low-risk, low risk**

A high-risk pregnancy.

He was /considered/designated/ at high risk of (acquiring) pneumonia.

They were subject to a high risk of pneumonia.

Compare: a heightened risk

role *n.* a part taken in an activity

A protective role for selenium against cancer has been postulated.

The immune system normally has a protective role against pathogenic organisms.

The role of this agent in controlling iron absorption is limited, /is uncertain/remains to be established.

This finding indicates a role for cell-mediated immunity in the pathogenesis of this disorder.

to play a role = to play a part

Compare: place

room *n.*

1. a division of a building

Blood flow in the thigh was recorded in a room at constant temperature.

Emergency conditions are handled in an emergency room.

Operating room, recovery room.

Compare: unit

2. scope, opportunity

There is no room for doubt in this diagnosis.

rotation *n.* a planned sequence

A rotation of hypnotics was used for their insomnia. A different hypnotic was given each night.

v. rotate

rough *adj.* approximate

A rough correlation, estimate.

round *n.* a series of calls by a doctor, a routine medical visit, especially in a hospital

A daily round is taken by the consultant staff of the unit.

route *n.*

1. a means of access

The route of transmission of a disease.

The safest and shortest route for the passage of the biopsy needle.

They had acquired the infection by the airborne route.

2. a route of administration of a drug

To administer a drug by the intramuscular, sublingual route.

3. a canal

Delivery by the vaginal route.

routine *adj.* ordinary, relating to established procedure

A routine weekly surveillance of transplantation recipients.

Routine medical insurance examination.

routine *n.* the usual procedure(s)

Hospital routine.

routinely *adv.* in a routine manner

Today, structures as small as the upper lip of the fetus are routinely studied by ultrasound.

rule out *vt.* to dismiss from consideration

The possibility of coronary obstruction was ruled out in diagnosis.

Compare: eliminate, exclude

run *vi. vt.*

1. to (cause to) flow

An infusion runs at a certain rate.

We run this infusion at a slow rate.

2. to carry out

We ran a battery of tests, serial blood cultures.

Note: She was running a high fever = She had a high fever.

rupture *vi. vt.* to (cause to) undergo a rupture

The fetal membranes had ruptured.

rupture *n.* the breaking or tearing of a tissue

The rupture of an aneurysm, membranes.

S

sacrifice *vt.* to give up for a purpose

To /sacrifice/write: kill/ experimental animals.

safe *adj.* free from danger or risk

A safe drug.

safeguard *n.* a safety measure

Urine tests were carried out as a safeguard against erroneous blood glucose readings.

safety *n.* the condition of being safe

The question of safety and toxicity in relation to drug efficacy.

The safety of this method has not been established in infants.

salient *adj.* striking, most important

The salient features of laboratory studies, of a history.

The (diagnostically) salient findings.

saltatory *adj.* (rare usage:) proceeding abruptly, not gradually

The saltatory deterioration of a patient.

Compare: precipitous

salvage *n.* the act of saving

Immediate surgical intervention offers the only hope of testicular salvage in cases of torsion.

v. salvage

sample *n.* a small part typically representing the whole

An unselected national sample of 892 children.

Blood samples were drawn at least 24 hours before catheterization.

Blood samples were /drawn/taken/ by standard venepuncture.

Urine samples were collected from patients.

Compare: specimen

sample *vt.* to collect a sample

Arterial blood was sampled from each baby.

satisfactorily *adv.* in a satisfactory manner

This mechanism has been explained satisfactorily.

satisfactory *adj.* fulfilling a need

The treatment of systemic sclerosis is not satisfactory.

saturate *vt.* to fill to capacity, to give as much as possible

He was saturated with large doses of adrenocortical steroids.

n. saturation

scale *n.* a graduated series or scheme of rank numbers or standards for measurement

Improvement of pain was assessed on a six-point scale (1 = pain entirely gone, 6 = much worse).

Patients were asked to describe their symptoms on a scale from 0 to 3, which corresponded to none, mild, moderate and severe.

scan *n.* an examination by or a product of scanning

A computed tomographic (CT) scan of the abdomen, a radioiodine scan of the thyroid gland detected, disclosed, revealed an abnormality.

Bone metastases were seen on bone scan.

Serial CT scans were obtained.

scan *vt.* to examine (for the presence of radioactive material)

To scan the brain

scar *n.* the connective tissue union produced by the edges of a wound

scarring *n.* scar formation

A barium meal examination showed duodenal scarring.

schedule *n.* a treatment regimen

Ketoprofen in two different dosage schedules was compared with aspirin.

scope *n.* the area (of the subject under discussion)

Paediatrics has enlarged its scope to include perinatology and adolescent medicine.

This discussion is beyond, outside, within, the scope of our study.

score *n.* a numerical record for the evaluation of the results of an examination

The Glasgow coma /score/scale/ is the sum of scores of clinical observations of eye (1–4 points), motor (1–6 points), and verbal (1–5 points) responses.

Their neurological disability score (a summed score of muscle strength, reflexes and sensory loss) decreased.

screen *vt.* to examine or test routinely an individual or a population group for the presence of a specific disease

Women of child-bearing age were screened for rubella antibodies.

screening *n.* a (mass) test or examination for detection of a disease

Screening examinations help in the early /discovery/identification/ of breast cancer.

search *n.* an act of searching

Asymptomatic bacteriuria should always prompt a thorough search for obstruction or prostatitis.

We evaluated 56 patients in search of a better method.

A search for literature; a search of the literature.

search *vt.* to look for, to examine carefully to find something

Scientists are searching for an AIDS vaccine.

To search the stool for a parasite.

secondarily *adv.* as a secondary phenomenon
The sellar region was involved secondarily by spread of tumour from nearby structures.

secondary *adj.* derived from something primary
A secondary (growth) = a metastasis.
These changes are secondary to other biochemical events.
Compare: primary

secrete *vt.* to produce a (usually liquid) substance (by a gland)
To secrete hormones.
n. secretion, *adj.* secretory
Compare: excrete; excretion; excretory

sedentary *adj.* relating to sitting
Sedentary life, work.

see *vt.*.
1. to examine, interview, meet
A doctor sees a patient.
2. to consult
A patient sees a doctor.
3. to observe
Dilated loops of bowel were seen on the radiograph.
Physiological changes were seen with this treatment.
Compare: find, note
4. to be seen = to occur
The syndrome is seen in children under 18 years of age.

seek *vt.* to try to obtain
To seek advice, consultation, medical help, treatment at a hospital.

seizure *n.* a sudden attack
The convulsive seizures of epilepsy.
Compare: attack, bout, fit

seldom *adv.* rarely
The results of this method have seldom been compared with those in untreated controls.

selected *adj.* chosen in preference
This treatment was used in selected patients.

self-limited, self-limiting *adj.* running a definite limited course
Q fever pneumonia is usually benign and self-limited.
Self-limiting bacteraemia.

send *vt.* to cause to go or to be taken
The sample was sent to our unit for examination.

sensation *n.* (a) direct feeling coming from the sense organs
To regain sensation in the legs.

sense *n.*

1. the faculty of a sense organ
The five senses are sight, hearing, taste, smell and touch.
2. appreciation
He had a poor sense of self.

sensitive *adj.*

1. capable of being stimulated
The tooth was sensitive to percussion.
2. responsive
Intracranial lymphomas may be highly sensitive to steroid therapy.
3. excessively susceptible
The patient was sensitive to penicillin.
4. capable of showing small differences
This test is a sensitive method for /detecting/the detection of/ many infections.

sensitize, sensitise *vt.* to make sensitive
The recipient had been sensitized to HLA antigens in the graft.
n. sensitization, sensitisation

separate *adj.* distinct, existing independently
Illustrations and tables should be put on separate sheets.
Two separate studies found that this risk increases with age.

separate *vi. vt.*

1. *vi. vt.* to (cause to) come apart
In genetic segregation the two alleles of each gene separate, so that they pass to different gametes.
The segregator was inserted into the urinary bladder to separate the cavity into two parts, so that the urine from each kidney could be collected separately.
2. *vt.* to keep apart
Bile canaliculi are always separated from the blood capillaries.
3. *vt.* to break or divide up into parts
These proteins can be separated on the basis of their molecular weight by chromatography.
4. *vt.* to isolate from a mixture
Fibrogen was separated from plasma by the addition of thrombin.
5. *vi.* to become divided or detached
The stump of the umbilical cord separates, leaving the umbilicus or 'navel' marking its place.
n. separation

separately *adj.* not together
To prevent individual bias in the tracing of the ventriculograms, two angiographers traced each study separately.
Compare: independently

sequel *n.* (*pl.* **sequels** or **sequelae**) a lesion or involvement due to injury or disease
Secondary lesions occurred as a sequel to raised intracranial pressure.
The sequelae of paralytic poliomyelitis are distinctive.
Compare: complication, consequence
sequence *n.* a series
A packeted sequence of 22 contraceptive tablets.
sequential *adj.* relating to a sequence
Sequential biopsy specimens.
serendipitous *adj.* accidental
The serendipitous discovery of a bone tumour.
Compare: chance, fortuitous, unexpected
serendipity *n.* the faculty of making discoveries by accident
Penicillin was discovered by serendipity.
series *n.* a group of patients in a study
A consecutive series of 11 patients with diabetes.
seropositive *adj.* positive in a serological test
He was seropositive for rheumatoid factor.
serve *vi.* to act
The transudate /served/acted/ as a medium for bacteria.
sessile *adj.* attached
Sessile tumours.
setting *n.* environment, circumstances
This method has not been applied in a clinical setting, /in/in the setting of/ a clinical trial.
settle *vi.* to subside (back to normal)
Even very high blood pressures can settle with rest.
Compare: reverse, revert, subside
set up *vt.* to design
To set up a study.
severe *adj.* very painful, serious
Severe disease, head injury, responses to a drug, symptoms.
The headaches were graded as severe, moderate or mild.
severity *n.* the quality or state of being severe
The severity of symptoms was assessed clinically.
shock *n.* collapse of vital processes and/or organs
He was admitted in shock.
Shock may ensue in severe cases of the disease.
Incipient ⟷ advanced shock.
Note: **shock** on its own means **hypovolaemic shock**
shortcoming *n.* defect
Prospective studies have the shortcoming that follow-up is incomplete.

Compare: defect, deficiency

short-lived *adj.* of short duration

Short-lived diuresis, drug efficacy, remission, symptoms.

Opposite: long-lived; prolonged

short-term *adj.* lasting a short time

Short-term treatment.

show *vt.*

1. to allow to be seen

These results show an excess of heavy consumers of alcohol among patients with stroke.

2. to state or to prove

The drug has been shown to be teratogenic in animals.

shunt *n.* a bypass, congenital or surgically created, between two vessels.

A cutaneous arteriovenous shunt.

v. shunt

shutdown *n.* suspension of function

Renal shutdown = inhibited renal tubular secretion.

sibling, sib *n.* a brother or a sister

The patient had two siblings; a brother aged 6 years and a sister aged 5 years.

Compare: offspring

sick *adj.*

1. affected with disease

Sick children.

2. nauseated

A seasick passenger.

sickness *n.*

1. a reaction of the body to pathogens or external circumstances

Compare: disease; illness

Sickness benefit.

2. nausea

side-effect, side effect *n.* an undesired effect produced by a therapeutic agent in a standard dose and form

A doctor may encounter, find, look for, observe, report side-effects.

A drug may /give rise to/induce/ side-effects.

Side-effects are acceptable, harmful, important, mild, moderate, serious, severe, trivial.

Side-effects may develop, emerge, occur with a drug.

Side-effects were fewer with drug B in this study.

The incidence of side-effects was /greater/higher ⟷ lower with this drug.

Compare: adverse effect, adverse reaction, toxic effect, undesired effect, untoward effect, unwanted effect

sign *n.* objective evidence of a disease

A favourable sign (such as loss of anorexia).

A physical sign = something detected on physical examination.

An ominous sign (in a moribund patient).

Compare: expression, feature, symptom

signal *vt.* to be a sign of

The disease is signalled by the abrupt onset of arterial hypertension.

Compare: herald, precede

significance *n.* the quality of being significant

The level of significance = the significance level.

The /significance/implications/ of these findings.

To reach statistical significance.

It is far more difficult to make an exact observation than to do a simple statistical test; and statistical significance does not necessarily imply clinical significance.

Note: For the sake of clarity, it might be preferable to use **significant** and **significance** about statistical significance only.

significant *adj.*

1. important

A significant finding.

2. statistically significant

The results were significant at the level of $p < 0.001$.

silent *adj.* symptom-free

A silent carrier of a disease.

Many urinary calculi are clinically silent.

The author found that 30% of myocardial infarcts recorded post-mortem had been clinically silent.

Compare: asymptomatic, dormant, inactive, latent, quiescent

similar *adj.* like, having resemblance to

Frozen semen gave similar fertilization rates to those obtained by freshly ejaculated semen.

Parental smoking habits were broadly, strikingly similar for all three groups of children.

Other adjectives expressing various aspects of similarity: comparable with/to, compatible with, consistent with, corresponding to, equal to, identical with, matched with, parallel to

similarity *n.* resemblance

A strong ($\longleftrightarrow$ weak) similarity was found between the two groups.

The groups bore a strong similarity.

Other nouns expressing various aspects of similarity: accord, agreement, conformity, consensus

similarly *adv.* in a similar manner

They were treated similarly to those with renal disease.

simple *adj.*

1. easy to understand or carry out

This method is easy to learn and technically simple.

2. free from complications

A /simple/closed/ fracture ⟷ a /compound/open/ fracture.

simulate *vt.* to have the outward qualities (signs and symptoms) of

Secondary syphilis may simulate the adenopathy of rubella.

Compare: masquerade, mimic

single-blind *adj.* of a clinical trial in which one participant, usually the subject rather than the observer or experimenter, does not know what treatment is being given at any specific time.

sinister *adj.* highly unfavourable

A low haemoglobin concentration in a severely dehydrated patient is a sinister finding.

site *n.* a place

A biopsy site, an injection site.

A drug acts at a receptor site

The easiest site for biopsy, injection.

The site of a lesion, the storage site of iron in the body.

sized *adj.* of a specified size

Small to moderately sized lesions.

slight *adj.* of low degree or amount

Slight/mild/ anaemia, haemorrhage.

Opposites: great, gross, severe, serious

slow *vt.* to make or become slower

To slow the heart rate of a patient.

The slowed conduction of a nervous impulse.

Compare: retard ⟷ accelerate, speed

smarting *n.* stinging pain

This adverse reaction was characterized by burning or smarting.

smear *n.* a preparation made for microscopic study by spreading material on a glass plate

A smear test.

Cervical smears revealed metaplastic cells.

Sputum smears for bacteria were unremarkable.

smear *vt.* to apply a smear

The pharyngeal swab was smeared on a microscopic slide.

so-called *adj.*

1. commonly named

The so-called type A personality.
2. incorrectly or tentatively named
So-called innocent heart murmurs.

source *n.* the point or place of origin
Eggs are a source of dietary cholesterol.

space *vt.* to give at intervals
The drug was given in equally spaced doses.

spare *vt.*
1. to keep from harming
No organ system is spared by this disease.
2. to relieve of the necessity of undergoing
Those patients free of chest pain were spared angiography.
3. to save
Potassium-/sparing/saving/ diuretics.
Compare: salvage

specific *adj.* particular, certain
Rheumatoid factors are not specific /for/to/ rheumatoid arthritis.
Opposite: non-specific

specimen *n.* a sample
Blood specimens were /collected/obtained/ for culture.

spectrum *n.* a (continuous) range
A spectrum of disease termed energy-protein malnutrition.
The /spectrum/range/ of activity of erythromycin is extensive.

speculate *vi.* to reason without knowing all pertinent facts
It is interesting to speculate on the possible mechanisms.

speculation *n.* an act or instance of speculating
The mechanisms responsible for insulin resistance during puberty are open to speculation.
This has raised the speculation/It has been suggested/ that the interactions of these cells serve as a surveillance mechanism.

speculative *adj.* characterized by speculation
Speculative estimates.

speed *n.* the rate of motion, growth, etc.
The children grew at normal speed.

speed *vt.* to give speed to
To speed the healing and resolution of symptoms.
Compare: accelerate

spill *vt.* to cause to run out of a container
To spill sugar and acetone in the urine.

spillage *n.* the act or process of spilling
The spillage of viable cells into the blood circulation.

split *vt.* to divide into separate parts
Papain splits the antibody molecule into two fragments.

Compare: break down

spontaneous *adj*. occurring without outside influence
Spontaneous mammary neoplasia in the dog.
Opposites: experimental, induced

spontaneously *adv*. without outside influence
The symptoms cleared, settled spontaneously.

sporadic *adj*. scattered; occurring irregularly
Sporadic cases of malaria.

spotlight *vt*. to call attention to
The use of hapten–protein conjugates has spotlighted the remarkable diversity of immune mechanisms.
Compare: highlight

spread *n*. the act or action of spreading
The /spread/transmission/ of a disease from A to B.
The mode of spread.

spread *vi*. *vt*. to (cause to) have a wider distribution
The disease is spread by sexual intercourse.
Compare: transmit

spurious *adj*. false
Spurious elevations of blood potassium levels.
Compare: false

spuriously *adv*. in a spurious manner
SGOT values may be elevated spuriously in acute liver damage.

stability *n*. the quality, state or degree of being stable
Emotional stability.
To achieve stability in a diabetic.

stabilization, stabilisation *n*. the process or result of stabilizing
The stabilization of a patient's condition.

stabilize, stabilise *vt*. to (cause to) become stable or keep in a stable condition
They were eventually stabilized on this dosage.
Compare: maintain

stable *adj*. not changing or easily changed, balanced
They were in a stable condition.

stage *n*. a phase
Response to treatment generally depends on the stage of disease.
The early ⟷ late stage of a disease.

stage *vt*. to determine the stage of a disease
We used laparotomy to stage patients with Hodgkin's disease.
They were clinically staged into one of four groups.

staging *n*. determination of the disease stage
Operative staging.

stain *n.* a microscopic laboratory test using a dye
A stain for tubercle bacilli was made on synovial fluid.
Bacteria can be recognized on Gram's stain.
Stains for tuberculosis were negative.

stain *vi. vt.*
1. to perform a stain
To stain a sample.
2. to become stained
This ulcer stains green with fluoroscein.

staining *n.* the procedure of performing a stain
To /do/carry out/ staining.

stand *vi.* of a fluid: to remain without flowing
The urine was allowed to stand.

standstill *n.* an arrest of function
Cardiac /standstill/arrest.

start *n.* a beginning
Three months after the start of treatment.

start *vt.* to begin (treatment)
They were started on indoramin, 25 mg twice daily.
A starting dose.

starvation *n.* a long-term deprival of food
Prolonged starvation.

starve *vi. vt.* to (cause to) be without food
A severely starved person.

state *n.* condition
Anxiety, disease, pain state.
Changes in the overall clinical state.
Patients in a steady state.
State-of-the-art equipment = equipment reflecting the latest
technical developments in the field.
The present state of cerebral microsurgery.
Compare: condition, status

status *n.* state or condition
The real status of the patient was determined before drug
therapy.
They had a low vitamin E status.

stay *n.* (temporary) residence
This treatment prolonged their inpatient stay.
A long-stay hospital.

stay *vi.* to reside (temporarily)
To stay a week in hospital.

step up *vt.* to increase, stimulate
To step up a dose.
Stepped-up cellular metabolism.

stiffness *n.* rigidity
Morning stiffness = stiffness on rising in the morning.

stillbirth *n.* the birth of a dead fetus or baby (after 28/52 gestation)
adj. stillborn ⟷ liveborn

stimulate *vt.* to excite functional activity with a stimulus
Cold air stimulates the nerves.
Excessive secretion of growth hormone stimulates the growth of bone.
Opposites: inhibit, suppress

stimulation *n.* the act or process of stimulating
The stimulation of a gland by a hormone.

stimulatory *adj.* pertaining to stimulation
The stimulatory action of a hormone.

stimulus *n.* (*pl.* **stimuli**) something that produces a reaction
Electrical, chemical, or physical stimuli.
This finding was a stimulus to research.
Compare: impetus

stool(s) *n.* faeces
To pass stools; the passage of stools.
Blood in the stool(s).

stop *vi. vt.* to discontinue
He stopped the drug after a month because of drowsiness.
Compare: cease, discontinue

storage *n.* the act of storing
Glycogen storage.

store *n.* a stock
Body iron stores; tissue stores of fat.
v. store

storm *n.* a violent disturbance, crisis
A thyroid storm = a critical stage of thyrotoxicosis.

stormy *adj.* marked by violent and disturbing symptoms
The course of the disease was stormy.

strain *n.*
1. excessive effort or exercise
v. strain
2. a breed of organisms
A bacterial strain.

stratify *vt.* to arrange in layers
The patients were stratified into three cigarette-consumption groups.
Compare: divide, group

strengthen *vt.* to make stronger
This contention was strengthened by new findings.
Compare: confirm, support

strenuous *adj.* demanding great effort

Strenuous exercise testing.

stress *n.* a physical, chemical or emotional strain

In international athletic events competitors impose on their bodies stresses and strains which are more severe than ever before.

To be under emotional stress.

To /tolerate/withstand/ stress.

Intrauterine stress due to rubella.

striking *adj.* attracting attention, easily perceivable

A striking correlation, difference.

The plasma cholesterol concentrations were lowered in a striking manner.

stringent *adj.* strict

Stringent criteria.

strong *adj.* not easily refuted

Strong evidence.

study *n.*

1. an investigation

To /carry out/conduct/make/undertake/ a study on/of/ a subject.

To /launch/initiate/ a study.

A study confirms, finds, something.

This phenomenon is under study.

Types of study: case-control, cohort study; cross-over, double-blind, randomized; single-blind, longitudinal $\longleftrightarrow$ cross-sectional, prospective $\longleftrightarrow$ retrospective.

2. an examination, a test

A microscopic study was made of posterior root ganglia.

An X-ray /study/examination/.

subdivide *vt.* to divide into smaller units

The classes were subdivided into three categories, subtypes.

n. subdivision

subject *adj.* tending or likely to have

Diabetics are subject to complications.

Compare: apt, prone, susceptible

subject *n.*

1. a theme or a topic

This enzyme has been the subject of considerable investigation.

A study on a subject.

2. an individual who undergoes an experiment or treatment

When the subject swallows, the sphincter segment relaxes normally.

subject *vt.* to cause to undergo

The rats were subjected to nephrectomy.

subjective *adj.* pertaining to the subject; perceived by the affected patient

Subjective assessment of symptoms, subjective symptoms.

subclinical *adj.* not detectable by clinical means

A subclinical disease.

Compare: dormant, inactive, latent, quiescent, silent

submit *vt.*

1. to make available

To submit a medical article for publication.

2. to subject or be subjected to

To submit a patient to treatment.

n. submission

subsequent *adj.* coming after something else, following

The symptoms were subsequent to hospital discharge.

Opposite: prior

subset *n.* a smaller unit

A subset of patients.

subside *vi.* to go back to the usual level

The drug was discontinued and her rash subsided.

n. subsidence

Compare: abate, decline, resolve, revert, settle

substantiate *vt.* to prove

A relationship between spontaneous abortion and physical trauma has not been substantiated.

Compare: establish

Note: to **substantiate** what has been **suggested**; to **confirm** what has been **proposed**.

substitute *n.* something substituted

An oral agent was used as a substitute for insulin.

substitute *vt.* to put in place of

Polyunsaturated fats should be substituted for animal fats.

n. substitution

Compare: replace

subtotal *adj.* less than total

A subtotal excision of a breast.

success *n.* the favourable outcome of an attempt

This method has met with limited success = Limited success has been obtained with this method.

The success rate of resuscitation.

Opposite: failure

successful *adj.* having success

The operation was successful in removing the foreign body.

succumb *vi.* to die of

He succumbed to encephalitis.

Note: **die of** is the plain verb.

suffer *vi. vt.*

1. *vt.* to experience an episode, an event

She suffered a miscarriage.

Some patients suffered paroxysms of coughing during the examination.

2. *vi.* to be subject to (often for a longer time)

A man /suffering from/with/ high blood pressure.

a sufferer (less formal) = **a patient**

sufficient *adj.* enough to meet a requirement

The reduction of unsaturated fats was sufficient to produce a fall in plasma cholesterol concentration.

adv. sufficiently

suggest *vt.*

1. to present a hypothesis

Enterogastric reflux of bile has been suggested as a cause of gastritis after operation.

The authors suggested that these responses become increasingly depressed with drug therapy.

Compare: hypothesize, postulate

2. to bring to mind by association

The diagnosis was suggested by the history and confirmed by laboratory investigations.

These surgical findings strongly suggested a diverticular abscess.

suggestion *n.*

1. something suggested

To confirm ⟷ refute a suggestion, to put forward a suggestion

2. a slight indication

The drug should be taken at the first suggestion of an attack.

suggestive *adj.* tending to suggest an idea

The presence of these factors is /highly/strongly/ suggestive of chronic glomerulonephropathy.

suitable *adj.* having the right qualifications

The patient was considered to be suitable for an operation.

n. suitability

Compare: appropriate; candidate

suited *adj.* suitable

These patients are well suited /for/to/ examination by tomography.

summarize, summarise *vt.* to make a (short) general account of

Table I summarizes our pathological findings.

This article summarizes the salient clinical applications of the method.

summary *n.* a section or paragraph of a paper giving the main points

To write a summary of a paper.

/In summary/in conclusion/, we observed that . . .

superimpose *vt.* to add to

Injury and disease superimpose their effects on the declining function of vital organs.

Primary liver cell carcinoma was superimposed on active cirrhosis.

Compare: complicate

superior *adj.*

1. higher in position

A strip of abdominal-wall skin immediately superior to the abdominal incision was excised.

2. better in effect, usefulness, etc.

Antimicrobial agents in combination are sometimes superior to a single agent.

superiority *n.* the fact or state of being superior

The superiority of one method over another.

supervene *vi.* to follow (as an additional unexpected development)

In this condition dementia supervenes unless the underlying condition is treatable.

n. supervention

Compare: complicate, superimpose

supervise *vt.* to direct

A medically supervised exercise programme.

Compare: control, monitor

supervision *n.* the act or action of supervising

Close supervision is required for hyperthyroid patients.

To be, keep, use under close medical supervision.

supplement *n.* an additional amount, given to correct a deficiency

He was given vitamin A supplements.

Compare: replacement

supplement *vt.* to make additions to

We supplemented endocardial resection /by/with/ an automatic cardioverter-defibrillator.

A diet supplemented /by/with/ fibre and fruit.

supplemental *adj.* serving to supplement

Patients receiving supplemental potassium.

supplementation *n.* addition of a supplement

Multivitamin supplementation may be needed.

Supplementation with calciferol.

supply *vt.* to provide

A tissue is supplied by blood vessels, nerves.

He was well supplied with tablets to relieve symptoms.

The drug is supplied in capsules, /as/in/ tablets.

supply *n.* stock, delivery

A rich supply of nerves = rich innervation.

Muscle haemoglobin supply.

Vascular supply.

support *n.* something that supports

Additional support to our theory has been derived, has come from other studies.

He received respiratory support by mechanical ventilation.

Support exists for both these schools of thought.

These findings lend support to our theory.

support *vt.*

1. to be in favour of, to corroborate

This view is supported by earlier studies.

Compare: confirm

2. to provide money

This work was supported by funding, a grant from the Hill Trust.

3. to help to maintain

To support pulmonary function.

Mechanically supported ventilation.

supportive *adj.* maintaining the well-being of a patient

Treatment is supportive and palliative in this disease; there is no specific cure.

suppress *vt.*

1. to eliminate or decrease

To suppress a headache with an analgesic.

To suppress the appetite.

To suppress fatigue.

Immunosuppressed ⟷ immunocompetent.

2. to inhibit a disease instead of curing it

To suppress an infection.

3. to stop a function

His thyroid function was suppressed.

adj. suppressive

Opposite: stimulate

suppression *n.* the act of suppressing, the state of being suppressed

The suppression of hormone production.

Opposite: stimulation

Note: immunosuppression

surgery *n.*
>1. treatment of disease by manual or operative procedures
>Surgery /of/on/ the stomach; surgery for peptic ulcer.
>Conservative, plastic, radical surgery.
>2. BE: the consulting room of a general practitioner
>The surgery was open from 4.30 to 6.30 p.m.
>Patients attend a doctor's surgery.
>A doctor treats his patients in his surgery.
>*Note*: the AE word is **office**.

surgical *adj.* relating to surgery
>A surgical instrument, method, operation.
>Surgical intervention, treatment.

surprising *adj.* unexpected
>A surprising finding.

surveillance *n.* a close watch
>Close clinical and x-ray surveillance after antibiotic treatment.
>To be under surveillance.

survey *n.* a general examination
>A survey of the literature.
>To carry out a skeletal survey in search of metastases.
>*Compare*: overview

survival *n.* continuation of life
>To decrease ⟷ improve, increase, prolong survival.
>Obstruction of airways threatens survival.
>The survival of the patient was the time from initial diagnosis
>of cancer until death.
>Survival after myocardial infarction, into adulthood.
>Long-term, disease-free survival.

survive *vi.* to remain alive (after)
>To survive an infarct.
>To survive to adolescence.

survivor *n.* one who survives
>A long-term survivor of cardiac arrest.
>Most patients were five-year survivors.

susceptible *adj.* easily influenced by or sensitive to
>Susceptible to infections.
>*n.* susceptibility
>*Other adjectives expressing various aspects of susceptibility*:
>apt, exposed, immune, prone, sensitive, subject to, vulnerable

suspect *vt.* to consider as probable
>He was strongly suspected of (having) spinal osteomyelitis.
>To suspect a disease from the patient's history.

suspected *adj.* considered as probable
>Patients with known or suspected infection.

suspicion *n*. the act of suspecting or the state of being suspected

Neurological abnormalities /aroused/raised/, heightened the suspicion of porphyria.

The clinical suspicion of this disease was low, supported by histological studies.

Various toxic chemicals have come under suspicion as a cause of this disease.

suspicious *adj*. arousing suspicion

Suspicious opaque bodies were noted in the region of the adrenal gland.

sustain *vt*.

1. to suffer

He had /sustained/incurred/ a myocardial infarction recently.

He sustained a compound fracture of the fibula, injuries of the spine.

2. to maintain a state, the effect of an action

An artificial organ was used to sustain terminal patients awaiting transplantation.

The effect of the drug was not /sustained/prolonged/.

Sustained fever = fever with temperature constantly above normal.

Sustained-release (SR) tablets.

swallowing *n*. taking (of food, etc.) through the mouth and oesophagus into the stomach

These vesicles cause pain on swallowing.

sweat(s) *n*. perspiration

Night sweats.

swell *vi*. to expand

The leg was swollen to the thigh.

swelling *n*.

1. the condition of being swollen, oedema

Facial swelling = the swelling of the face.

2. something that is swollen

A swelling on the face.

swing *n*. fluctuation

Swings in plasma glucose after a meal

Compare: fluctuation, oscillation

symptom *n*. subjective evidence of a (particular) disease

To have, show symptoms of a disease.

To /cause/produce/ symptoms.

To /abate/ease/reduce/relieve/ ⟷ aggravate symptoms.

Abatement/relief/ ⟷ aggravation of symptoms.

These symptoms are brought on by mastication.

These symptoms /arise/come on/ abruptly.

Without symptoms = symptom-free.

symptomatic *adj.*

1. showing symptoms (of)

If the disease becomes symptomatic, surgery is necessary.

Patients persistently /symptomatic of/showing symptoms of/ cardiac arrhythmias.

Opposite: asymptomatic, silent

2. relating to or according to symptoms.

Symptomatic relief = relief of symptoms.

Symptomatic treatment.

symptomatically *adv.* according to symptoms

He was treated symptomatically.

syndrome *n.* traditional definition: a combination of signs and symptoms; current definition: a condition which is defined and characterized by a complex aetiology, involvement of several organs with varied symptoms

Parkinsonian syndrome = postencephalitic syndrome, characterized by muscular rigidity, slow involuntary tremor, festinating gait, etc.

systemic *adj.* involving the whole body

Systemic circulation.

Note: **systematic** = using a regular plan or method.

T

table *n.* a systematic display of data, usually in columns
Table I shows the distribution of patients according to diagnosis.
The results are presented in Table I = simply: Table I shows . . .
As can be seen from Table I = simply: Table I shows that . . .
Best used with active verbs:
Table I compares, details, gives, shows, etc.

tablet *n.* a solid block of medicine; informally: a pill
Sustained-release tablets, scored tablets.
The drug is available as sugar-coated 0.1 mg tablets.

tabulate *vt.* to illustrate by means of a table
The results are tabulated for three five-year groups.

tailor *vt.* to adapt to suit some specific purpose
The dosage must be tailored to (the needs of) each (individual) patient.

take *vt.*
1. to ingest a drug
Those who took this drug did not develop symptoms.
2. to adhere
Allografts took readily on the well-vascularized granulations.

take in *vt.* to eat, ingest
Men tend to take in more animal fat than women.
n. intake

take up *vt.* to absorb
Creatinine is taken up from the bloodstream by the muscles.
n. uptake

tantamount *adj.* equivalent
Relapse was considered tantamount to a complete failure of treatment.

target *n.* an object, an organ or area at which an action or development is directed
Different antipsychotic drugs affect target symptoms selectively.
To direct antibodies at a target.

target *vt.* to make a target of
A cytotoxic agent is targeted to metastatic disease.
These antibodies target the cell membrane.

technique *n.* a method
To use a technique for a purpose.

temper *vt.* to adjust to the requirements of a situation
Treatment of the mother was tempered by concern for the fetus.

temporary *adj.* lasting for a limited period
The treatment gave only temporary relief.
Opposites: permanent; prolonged

tendency *n.* a natural likelihood of developing
Adenocarcinoma has a tendency to recur systematically.
Obese persons have a tendency to retain water.
They developed a tendency for convulsions.
Compare: inclination, trend

tender *adj.* sensitive, painful (in response to being examined)
The abdomen was moderately tender to palpation.

tenderness *n.* the quality of being tender
Mild, diffuse tenderness to palpation.
n. tenderness

tenuous *adj.* weak, flimsy
Tenuous emotional stability.
Tenuous evidence.

tenuously *adv.* on weak evidence
Pyelonephritis in pregnancy has been tenuously associated with prematurity and neonatal death.

term *n.*
1. a period of time
The treatment improved the appetite of these patients in the short term.
The drug was administered short term ⟷ long term.
adj. long-term, short-term, medium-term
2. the time at which childbirth usually occurs
Birth was at term.
Ten pregnancies went to term in eight women.
The diabetic mother was allowed to go to term.
adj. preterm, full-term, post-term

terminal *adj.* of an illness that will end in death
Terminal cancer = cancer without recovery.
The terminal ward.
Compare: end-stage

terminate *vi. vt.*
1. *vt.* to bring to an end
To terminate medication, a postdate pregnancy.
2. *vi.* to come to an end
Her polyarteritis /terminated/simply: ended/ in cardiac failure.
Compare: abort, cease, discontinue, end, stop

termination *n.* an end, the act of termination

The termination of a disease attack, pregnancy.

test *n.* an examination or investigation

To /do/make/conduct/carry out/ a test /on/in/ a patient, on a specimen.

To do a specific test for glucose.

The Kahn test is done on the blood.

Analysis of the data by Student's *t* test.

She had normal results on liver-function tests.

She showed marked toxicity on the routine haematological test.

An informative, equivocal test.

test *vt.* to make a test

The drug was tested against another drug.

The urine specimen was tested for protein and blood.

testimony *n.* evidence

The high death rate is powerful testimony to the lethal nature of global brain anoxia and ischaemia.

theatre *n.* an operating room

He was taken from the admitting room direct to theatre (BE).

He was taken to /surgery/the (operating) theater (AE).

theory *n.* a formulated hypothesis

To advance, present, propose a theory on a phenomenon.

To disprove, prove, test a theory

adj. theoretical

theorize, theorise *vi.* to present a theory

The authors /theorized/plainly: suggested/ that these mechanisms inhibit the growth of neoplastic cells.

therapeutic *adj.* of or relating to treatment

Side-effects may occur even with the usual therapeutic dose.

The /therapeutic outcome/result of the treatment.

Compare: diagnostic

therapy *n.* treatment of disease

To apply, give radiotherapy.

To direct therapy at correcting a dysfunction.

To /start/institute/ therapy.

He recovered with this therapy.

Oral infections should receive specific therapy.

Many-faceted, protracted, vigorous therapy.

thereafter *adv.* (simply:) then, afterwards

think *vt.* to consider

Amniocentesis was thought necessary.

thorough *adj.* carried through completely

A thorough abdominal examination showed nothing abnormal.

thready *adj.* (especially about pulse:) weak

The pulse may be thready in pulmonary oedema.

threat *n.* something that presents a danger

The disease /represents/poses/ a threat to life = It is potentially fatal.

A life-threatening emergency.

threshold *n.* a value above which a phenomenon will take place and is perceived

Cigarette smoking causes a significant fall in the threshold for ventricular fibrillation.

Some physicians have a low threshold for altering treatment.

thrive *vi.* to develop well and be healthy

The child was thriving.

throughput *n.* the number of patients treated

The throughput of patients in the x-ray department.

titrate *vt.* to determine by small changes

The dose of the drug should be titrated against the effect (starting with the lowest effective dose and increasing slowly with increments not exceeding the starting dose, until the desired response is attained or unacceptable side-effects occur).

n. titration

to *prep.* referring to a range of degree, values, etc.

Haemolysis is mild to severe in this condition.

toilet *n.*

1. urination and defaecation

He rested in bed, apart from going to the toilet.

2. cleansing

Wound toilet.

tolerance *n.*

1. the need to increase the dose progressively to produce the effect initially brought about by smaller amounts

Tolerance to the drug emerged.

2. the capacity to endure without adverse effects

To acquire tolerance to a drug without ill effect.

Exercise tolerance.

3. specific immunological non-reactivity

To induce tolerance to an antigen.

Opposite: sensitivity

tolerant *adj.*

1. able to tolerate or endure without ill effect

He was tolerant of penicillin.

The body is less tolerant of osmotic pressure changes.

2. immunologically non-reactive

The recipient was made tolerant to the transplantation antigens present in the donated organ.

tolerate *vt.* to endure without ill effect

The drug is well ⟷ poorly tolerated at this dosage.

The patients tolerated the procedure well.

tool *n.* a useful aid

A valuable diagnostic, investigative tool.

This test is valuable only as a research tool.

total *n.* or *adj.* (the) whole

A total of 96 untreated cases = plainly: 96 untreated cases.

toxic *adj.* poisonous

Toxic effect = an adverse effect produced by a therapeutic agent given in overdose.

toxicity *n.* the quality of being poisonous

To produce toxicity.

transform *vi. vt.* to (cause to) change (completely)

These cells transformed nitroblue tetrazolium from colourless to deep blue during phagocytosis.

T memory cells will transform into lymphoblasts.

transformation *n.* a (complete) change in form

The transformation of normal cells into malignant cells.

transfuse *vt.* to transfer a fluid (e.g blood) into a blood vessel

He was transfused with 4 units of blood.

n. transfusion

Compare: infuse

transient *adj.* lasting only for a short time

A transient complication, fever.

Compare: acute, chronic; intermittent, remittent, temporary

transit *n.* a passage

Delayed intestinal transit time.

translation *n.* transformation

The translation of genetic material into chromosomes.

v. translate

transmission *n.* spread

Modes of transmission: genetic transmission, hand-to-hand transmission, man-to-man transmission.

Transmission from inhalation of droplets.

transmit *vt.* to spread

The disease is transmitted by personal contact, by such objects as combs and hats.

A sexually transmitted disease (formerly: venereal disease, a venereally transmitted disease).

Transmitted from rodent to man.

adj. transmittable, transmissible

transplant *n.*

1. the transfer of tissue = transplantation

Ten weeks after (the) transplant the marrow returned to its pretransplant state.

2. something transplanted = a graft

transplant *vt.* to move an organ from one part of the body to another, or from one person or animal to another in a transplant operation

The author transplanted parathyroid glands into rats.

n. transplantation

trauma *n.* a physical or mental injury

He /sustained/suffered, had a severe injury, trauma of the brain.

The trauma of the death of a near relative.

traumatic *adj.* pertaining to trauma, causing trauma

Cystoscopy may be traumatic in men.

Traumatic life experiences.

travel *vi.* to move

An infection may travel along the artery and become an abscess in the thigh.

treat *vt.* to try to cure, to care

To treat a patient for renal failure by haemodialysis.

Lymphomas are usually treated /by/with/ surgery.

treatable *adj.* capable of being treated

Treatable endocrine disorders.

Opposites: intractable, untreatable

Compare: curable

n. treatability

treatment *n.*

1. the management and care of a patient to cure a disease or its symptoms

To extend treatment/beyond/after/ healing.

To direct treatment at an organ, at high-risk groups, at preserving cells.

To give treatment to a patient, to provide treatment for a patient, for a disease.

To start ⟷ /stop/discontinue/withdraw/, withhold; continue, alter treatment.

(Empiric) symptomatic treatment; injudicious treatment.

He was /under/receiving/ treatment with the drug.

He showed improvement while on treatment.

The treatment induced remission.

The benefits ⟷ risks of treatment.

Compare: care, management, therapy

2. a substance or a method used in treating a patient

Penicillin is the treatment of choice in this disease.

Compare: remedy

trend *n.* a general direction or course of development

A trend to blurred vision was apparent with this drug.

Compare: tendency

trial *n.* a test

To /do/conduct/mount/ a trial.

To /carry out/conduct/ a trial of a drug in patients.

To accept patients into a trial, to admit patients to a trial ⟷
to exclude from a trial, to select patients for (inclusion in) a
trial.

Six patients completed the trial.

Ten patients defaulted in the trial, withdrew from the trial.

This drug is under trial.

A blind, double-blind, cross-over, (case-, placebo-) controlled, randomized, therapeutic trial.

trigger *n.* a precipitating factor

To act as a trigger of a disease.

trigger *vt.* to start, to set off

These attacks may be triggered by several factors.

To trigger a hypersensitivity reaction, an immune response.

Compare: induce, precipitate

trivial *adj.* not important

A trivial symptom.

troublesome *adj.* annoying

Aerophagy is a troublesome habit.

trough *n.* a low point

A trough in the blood insulin concentration.

Opposite: peak

true *adj.*

1. possessing the basic characteristic of

True precocious puberty.

True ulcer relapse rate (including silent ulcers).

2. in accordance with facts

Raised urinary concentrations of adrenaline usually indicate
an intra-adrenal tumour. This was true of our patients.

Compare: imaginary, real

try *vt.* to study in a trial

Treatment with transfer factor is being /tried/studied/ by this
research team.

unanimity *n.* agreement

There is no unanimity about whether this factor is abnormal in hypertensive patients.

adj. unanimous

Compare: agreement

unavailable *adj.* not available

Blood pressure data were unavailable in these patients (=There were no records of their blood pressure readings).

unaware *adj.*

1. not aware

We /are unaware/clearer: do not know/ of any reports of controlled trials on this subject.

2. blinded

Serum samples were coded so that laboratory personnel were unaware of study group assignment.

uncomplicated *adj.* without complications

Uncomplicated meningioma.

under *prep.*

1. beneath

Thin sections were examined under the electron microscope.

2. subject to

He was under medication.

Laparoscopy was carried out under general anaesthesia.

This phenomenon is under study.

underdiagnose *vt.* to diagnose in inadequate numbers; to overlook, miss cases

Accidental hypothermia has been an underdiagnosed condition for centuries.

undergo *vt.* to experience

These cells had undergone viral transformation.

He underwent adrenalectomy for Cushing's syndrome.

underlie *vi.* to be the basic cause of

Circadian biological rhythms may underlie nocturnal asthma.

underlying *adj.*

1. located under

The premature infant tends to have thin, pink skin through which the underlying veins are easily seen.

Opposite: overlying

2. basic, primary

Most patients with true haemoptysis have an underlying pulmonary infarct.

The mechanisms underlying these disturbances.

The underlying disease, mechanism.

underreferral *n.* insufficient referral

Underreferral of patients for dialysis.

understanding *n.* comprehension, knowledge

An understanding of this phenomenon has evolved rapidly over the past decade.

Our understanding of this phenomenon is progressing.

Rational diagnosis of the disease requires an understanding of the underlying endocrinological factors.

This information should lead to a clearer understanding, an improved understanding of this phenomenon.

Advances in our understanding of this disease.

According to current understanding.

Compare: knowledge

understood *adj.* fully apprehended

This phenomenon is not clearly, /completely/fully/ understood.

This phenomenon is /imperfectly/incompletely/ not fully/only partially/, poorly understood.

Compare: ill-understood, misunderstood

undertake *vt.* to perform

To undertake an investigation, a procedure, research, a study, a survey, a trial.

underusage *n.* inadequate usage

The underusage of a drug.

underway, under way *adv.* in progress

Studies are /underway/in progress/ to investigate this phenomenon.

undesirable *adj.* unwanted

Excessive doses of the drug have undesirable effects.

undue *adj.* excessive

Diagnostic errors may result from/undue reliance/over-reliance/ on laboratory data.

Undue susceptibility to infections.

unequivocal *adj.* leaving no room for doubt

Unequivocal radiological evidence of pyelonephritis.

Unequivocal test results.

Compare: clear

unequivocally *adv.* clearly

They died of unequivocally natural causes.

uneventful *adj.* marked by absence of disease or complications

An uneventful appendicectomy had been performed under ether.

He had an uneventful childhood.
The postoperative course was uneventful.
Compare: unremarkable

unexpected *adj.* not expected
adv. unexpectedly

unexplained *adj.* without any apparent cause
Sudden unexplained death, unexplained fever.
Compare: unknown

unfortunately *adv.* it is unfortunate (that)
The haemolysis slowly subsided and the jaundice improved; unfortunately, the mental confusion persisted.

unfruitful *adj.* unrewarding
Laparoscopy was /unfruitful/unrewarding/.
Compare: disappointing, frustrating

uniform *adj.* having an unchanging pattern
There was a uniform change in all patients.
Compare: consistent

uniformly *adv.* in a uniform pattern
In these infections concurrent pulmonary disease is common but not uniformly present.
Compare: consistently

unique *adj.* being the only one of its type
Increase in contractility is unique to dobutamine among these drugs.

unit *n.*
1. a department in a hospital or other institution
She was transferred to the intensive care unit.
To work on the intensive care unit
2. a measure
Fluorescence data were expressed in arbitrary units (AU) per milligram of collagen.

unknown *adj.* not known
A disease of unknown aetiology, fever of unknown origin.
The cause of this cardiomyopathy remains completely unknown.
The disease may develop insidiously and unknown to the patient.
For reasons unknown.
Compare: unexplained

unlikely *adj.* improbable
This treatment is unlikely to preserve the function of the deep venous valves.

unobtainable *adj.* not obtainable
Blood pressure was unobtainable in two patients.

unreliable *adj*. not dependable

Physical examination has been shown to be unreliable in detecting retractile testes.

unremarkable *adj*. without any medical data worthy of attention

An unremarkable appendicectomy.

He had an unremarkable childhood.

Compare: uneventful

unresponsive *adj*. not responsive

Unresponsive to treatment.

unrewarding *adj*. not producing the desired result

Surgical exploration of the gland was unrewarding.

Compare: disappointing, unfruitful

unsatisfactory *adj*. not satisfactory

Radionuclide imaging is unsatisfactory for the diagnosis of chronic cholecystitis.

The therapy of this disease remains unsatisfactory (surgical procedures are not successful and medical treatment is limited).

unsuccessful *adj*. not successful

Surgery may be unsuccessful in such cases.

untoward *adj*. undesirable

An untoward effect = a side-effect.

unwanted *adj*. undesirable

Placebos also may cause unwanted effects.

It is not only faulty contraception which leads to unwanted children.

Compare: undesirable

unwell *adj*. in poor health (especially for a short time)

Beta-blockers often make patients feel unwell and a few extremely ill.

upset *n*. a disturbance (usually slight)

The usual constitutional upsets were minimal.

upset *vt*. to disturb

High doses of steroids always upset diabetic control.

upsurge *n*. a rapid increase

An upsurge in (the incidence of) melanoma.

v. surge (up)

uptake *n*.

1. absorption and incorporation of a substance into a living organism

The drug increases glucose uptake in the forearm muscles.

The uptake of radiolabelled antibody into tumours.

Increased ⟷ suppressed uptake.

2. acceptance

The national uptake of pertussis immunization declined.

usage *n.* simply: use

use *n.* the act of using; the state of being used

The use of a method, treatment.

To put a drug to clinical use, to take into use.

use *vt.* to put into action or service

To use a method, treatment.

useful *adj.* valuable

Laboratory studies are useful in these patients, in diagnosing arthritis.

A /useful/valuable/ treatment.

usefulness *n.* value

These drugs have limited /usefulness/briefly: value.

usher in *vt.* to precede

The icteric phase of hepatitis is /ushered in/simpler: preceded/ by the appearance of dark urine.

using *prep.* by, by means of

utilize, utilise *vt.* (simply:) to use

This investigation /utilized/simply: used/ human proteins.

V

valid *adj.*

1. (of a reason or an argument) having a strong firm basis
Parkinson's observations are still valid.
2. having value, objectively acceptable
A valid animal model for study.
Compare: relevant, useful

validate *vt.* to confirm
At the one-year follow-up, claims of abstinence from smoking
were /validated/simply: confirmed/ by measurement of expired
air/carbon monoxide concentrations.
To /validate/confirm/ a hypothesis.
Compare: confirm, support

valuable *adj.* having beneficial qualities
This treatment is valuable for patients with Cushing's syn-
drome.
Compare: beneficial, helpful, useful

value *n.*

1. usefulness
The long-term value of this treatment is /questionable/doubt-
ful/ $\longleftrightarrow$ well-established.
2. a specific numerical record of an amount
Laboratory values.

valueless *adj.* without value
Endocrine treatments are valueless in this disease.
Compare: useless

variability *n.* changeability
There has been considerable variability in these studies =
Their results have been divergent.

variable *adj.* changeable
The course of diabetes is extremely variable.
The disorder progresses at a variable rate.
The results of immunological studies of transplant-associated
lymphomas have been variable.
This treatment has been used with variable success.

variance *n.* at variance = not in agreement
Our results are at variance with those of Hill *et al*.
Compare: disagreement

variation *n.* an instance of varying
The variations between our results and those of others.
Compare: difference

various *adj.* of different kinds, diverse
Various topical treatments are used in psoriasis.

vary *vi.* to show change
The potency of the drug varies widely among patients.

varying *adj.* showing change in a continuous process
He showed varying degrees of hypertension.
These studies have given varying results.

vector *n.* a carrier of a disease
These men act as vectors of infection from one community to another.

vehicle *n.* something used to pass on or spread something else
Soft lenses are used as vehicles for delivering topical medications to the eyes.

via *prep.* through
Haemodialysis via a subclavian catheter.

viability *n.* capacity for living
The viability of a fetus; the viability of malaria parasites.
Transplant viability
adj. viable

viable *adj.* capable of existing and developing
At 28 weeks the fetus is viable, that is, capable of living a separate existence from the mother.
Viable leukaemia cells.

view *n.*
1. opinion
Many investigations favour, support ⟷ refute this view.
This view has been challenged in a recent study.
To take a strong view on something.
2. visual aspect (in x-ray studies)
Lateral views were /obtained/taken/ of each foot.
This view showed calcification in 10 patients.
This was detected /in/on/ lateral view.
3. in view of = in consideration of
This incidence is low in view of the long trial period.
4. with a view to = with the intention of
The operation was carried out /with a view to alleviating/ briefly: to alleviate/ these symptoms.

vigilance *n.* alertness
Clinical vigilance is necessary in this treatment.
adj. vigilant

vision *n.* sight
Normal vision; low vision – blindness.

visit *n.* a formal call
A patient makes a visit to a clinic for a symptom, a disease.

Laboratory studies were carried out at each visit to the clinic.

The index visit is followed by follow-up visits.

Compare: attendance

visualization, visualisation *n.* the process of visualizing

Cholangiography showed visualization of the bile ducts with non-visualization of the gall bladder.

X-ray visualization of intrathoracic structures.

visualize, visualise *vt.* to make visible by surgery or by a radiopaque substance followed by roentgenography

To visualize /by/with/ ultrasound and arteriography.

visually *adv.* with the naked eye

To examine a sample visually for haemoglobin.

volunteer *n.* a person who offers himself for a service of his own free will

Healthy volunteers provided blood samples for the study.

v. volunteer

vulnerable *adj.* easily damaged or injured

To be /vulnerable/plainly: susceptible/ to a disease.

The skin may be vulnerable to sunlight.

n. vulnerability

Compare: susceptible

W

waking *adj*. relating to the time of being awake
During waking hours and at night.
wane *vi*. to decrease gradually (in intensity)
Immunity may wane.
Interest in this disease has waned.
Opposite: wax
Compare: decline, decrease
ward *n*. a hospital unit
A patient /in/on/ this ward.
In a hospital ward, clinic.
warm *vt*. to make warm, heat gently
The drug was warmed to body temperature.
warrant *vt*. to justify (supported by the authority of precedent, experience or logic)
The symptoms warranted an operative procedure.
The use of heparin appeared warranted.
Compare: justify
washout *n*. elimination of a drug from the body
The trial was preceded by a washout period when no drugs were allowed.
wash out *vt*. to wash free of an unwanted substance
His eyes were washed out with an isotonic saline solution.
Compare: flush
waste *vi*. to lose strength
Muscle masses waste in starvation.
The patient was toxic, wasted, and seriously ill.
watch *n*. close observation
A careful watch should be kept on these patients for urinary infection.
Compare: alert, surveillance
watch *vt*. to keep under close observation
We watched him closely for signs of circulatory overload.
Compare: monitor, observe
way *n*. a manner or method
Subcutaneous heparin appears to be a safe way of anticoagulation during pregnancy.
wax *vi*. to increase
The waxing and waning of the peripheral pulse, symptoms
Opposite: wane
weaken *vi*. *vt*. to (cause to) become weak or weaker

A heart weakened by infection.
Compare: attenuate, blunt, compromise, cripple, debilitate, depress

wean *vt.* to cause to give up (gradually)
The asthmatic patient was weaned /from/off/ the ventilator.
To wean a patient from a drug (treatment).
To wean an infant (from mother's milk).
Compare: to withdraw

wear *vt.* to use
These women were wearing an intrauterine device.

wear off *vi.* disappear gradually
The effects of the drug will wear off after two to three days.

weigh *vt.* to consider (carefully)
Potential benefits (of the drug) must be weighed against the risks of abuse.

welfare *n.* well-being, comfortable life
Health has a fundamental influence on human welfare.

well *adj.* in good health
He appeared well on examination.
A well-baby clinic (especially AE).
Well individuals.

well-being *n.* good health
He survived with relative well-being for over a year.
The atrial extrasystoles impaired his well-being.

whereby *rel. adv.* by which
This is a technique /whereby/usually: by which/ the anaesthetist can assess several changes.

whether *conj.* indicating alternatives
Ketosis leads to acidosis, whether the ketosis is due to diabetes, to starvation or a high-fat diet.

wide *adj.* widespread
The wide use of a drug, a method.
This method has achieved wide acceptance.
Compare: extensive

with *prep.*
1. in the use of
This effect is often seen with penicillin.
2. suffering from, affected by
Patients with diabetes.
3. as a result of
Medical problems can arise with the expansion of pulmonary gas.
4. in proportion to
The incidence of cirrhosis increases with age.

withdraw *vi. vt.*
    1. *vt.* to take or draw away
    High-protein foods were withdrawn from his diet.
    The drug was withdrawn because of severe side-effects.
    Two patients were withdrawn from the study because of adverse effects.
    2. *vt.* to collect a sample
    Blood samples were withdrawn by routine venepuncture.
    3. *vi.* to detach oneself
    He had withdrawn from social interaction.

withdrawal *n.* an act or process of withdrawing
    Side-effects led to the withdrawal of the drug.
    Withdrawal from barbiturates.
    Withdrawal symptoms.
    The withdrawal of a blood specimen.
    Social withdrawal = active avoidance of verbal or non-verbal interaction with other people, or of being in the physical presence of other people (WHO 2).

withhold *vt.* to refrain from giving
    Antibiotics were withheld.
    We withheld this information, because it might have damaged the patient.

within *prep.* before a certain time has elapsed
    They relapsed within five months of stopping the drug.

within-patient *adj.* between-patient
    A within-patient comparison.
    Compare: interpatient

work *n.*
    1. a study, studies
    A recent work suggesting a relation between motor neuron disease and heavy metals.
    All the published work relating to this method.
    Work in London has shown that . . .
    2. workload
    Angina pectoris occurs when cardiac work and myocardial oxygen demand exceed the ability of the coronary system to supply oxygen.

worker *n.* a research worker
    His article aroused controversy among American workers.
    Brown and co-workers (= Brown *et al.*, Brown and colleagues).

workload *n.* the amount of work to be done
    Cardiac workload = workload imposed on the heart.
    Compare: burden, load, overload

work-up (AE) *n.* examination and investigations
    Gastrointestinal work-up was diagnostic.
work up (AE) *vt.* to examine and investigate a patient in order to
    arrive at a diagnosis
worsen *vi.* to deteriorate
    His condition worsened suddenly.
    The worsening of a condition, disease, patient.
    Compare: deteriorate
worthwhile *adj.* useful
    The use of the drug was worthwhile.

X

x-ray *n*.
1. electromagnetic radiation
2. x-ray examination

A plain x-ray examination of the abdomen provides an accurate assessment of spleen size and reveals opaque gall stones.

Chest x-ray films were obtained for the neonates.

The lesion was discovered on x-ray films of the spine.

x-ray *vt*. to examine by x-rays

The leg was x-rayed.

Y

yield *n*. result(s)

Diagnostic yield.

yield *vt*.
1. to produce

The tests /yielded/gave/ information, results.

The urine samples /yielded/showed/ cytomegalovirus.
2. to respond to treatment

The infection yielded to the treatment.

Compare: respond

Z

zero *n*. 0, nought

At time zero he started exercising.

A zero-hour reading.

Compare: baseline

Appendix

A GUIDE TO CLARITY

How can you make your words and sentences clearer, shorter and more concise? The following is a suggested list of improvements. However, these suggestions do not apply to all communicative situations, and they should therefore be applied cautiously. Some authors might claim that they use some of the words and phrases in the left column, because they want to avoid monotony. Read carefully through your paper. If you find any of the words and phrases listed here, consider whether your text could be improved with equivalents suggested in the right column.

according to our studies	our studies show that
accordingly	so, therefore
advantageous	helpful, useful
aid	help
aliquot	portion, sample
amount:	
a /considerable/large/ amount of	much
a /decreased/smaller/ amount of	less
an /increased/larger/ amount of	more
analysis: in the last analysis	in the end
anticipate	expect
appropriate	(sometimes:) suitable
approximately	(shorter:) about
are of the same opinion	agree
as already stated	miss out?
as can be seen from Fig. 1	Fig. 1 shows that
as follows	:
as far as calcium is concerned, it was	calcium was
as for Hill's study, it was	Hill's study was
as of now	now
as shown in Fig. 1	Fig. 1 shows
As regards/regarding/ molars, they are	molars are
assist	help
at some future time	later, in the future
at the present moment	now
author(s), the present author(s)	I/we?
avail oneself of	use
aware: to be aware of	know
awareness	knowledge
basis: on an outpatient basis	as an outpatient

be of assistance	help, be helpful
beneficial	helpful, useful
case (if a person is meant:)	patient, subject
clinical	miss out?
clinical entity	disease? symptom?
colour: red in colour	red
commence	start, begin
comparatively better	better
compared: better compared with	better
concerning these patients, it was found that	miss out!
considerably	miss out?
created the possibility	enabled (a person)
	permitted, allowed (an action)
data	facts, findings, results
date: to date	so far
deleterious	harmful
demonstrate	show
detrimental	harmful
disclose	show
disease entity	disease
disease process	disease
due to	because of, owing to
due to the fact that	because
during the time that	while
elevated	raised, higher, more
employ	use?
encountered	met, found
encountered frequently	common
engaged: to be engaged in the study of	to study
entail	involve?
establish	find out, show
even if	although
event: in the event of, in the event that	if
evidence, evince	show
exhibit	show
existing symptoms	symptoms
extremities	hands, feet, etc.
fairly	miss out!
females	women
fewer in number	fewer
following the operation	after the operation?

for the reason that	because
greater in number	more
humans	man, human beings
hypothesize	suggest?
if conditions are such that	if
in a few cases	sometimes
in all cases	always, invariably
in excess of	more than, greater than
in order to	to
in regard	
in relation to	
in respect of	use a suitable
in terms of	preposition,
in the case of	e.g. in, for, about,
in the context of	on
in the event of	
in the presence of	
in the present communication	here, in this paper, letter, etc.
in the event that	if
in view of the fact that	because
indicate	show
infant	(general meaning:) baby, child
irrespective of	whether or not,
it has been known a long time that	miss out!
it is a well known fact that	miss out!
it is interesting to note that	miss out!/ interestingly
it is often the case that	often
it is possible that	possibly
it is recognized that	miss out!
it should be emphasized that	miss out?
it may be said that	possibly, perhaps
it may well be that	possibly
it seems to the present writer that	I think; it seems that
it will be seen from Table I	Table I shows
it would thus appear that	apparently
large in size	large
length: of such length that	so long that
- level	concentration?
limbs, lower	legs
limbs, upper	arms
literature	reports?

made an analysis	analysed, assayed
major	large, main, important
majority of	most
males	men
manifest	show
material	study, population, patients?
meaningful	miss out?!
mental patients	psychiatric patients
multiple	several, many
number: a large number of	many
number: a number of	several
number: a small number of	few
owing to the fact that	because
parameter (if not a specific meaning)	criterion, factor, index, measure, value, variable?
perform	do?
pertaining	on, of, about
practically	almost
present in association with	associated
present in only small numbers	scanty, few, rare
present: presents a similar picture to	resembles
prior to	before?
proportion: a proportion of	some
proportion: a large proportion of	many, most
question: the cells in question	these cells
quite	miss out!
rather	miss out!
regime	regimen
relatively	miss out?
render	make
result: as a result of	because of
result: with the result that	so that
reveal	show
roentgenographic study	x-ray study
sacrifice (experimental animals)	kill
serve: it serves the function of transport	it transports
shape: round in shape	round
significantly (if not statistically:)	appreciably, markedly, noticeably?
size: small in size, of small size	small

skin rash	rash
sophisticated	advanced, complex, new
spectrum	range
subsequent to	after, following
subsequently	then, after(wards), later
terminate	end, stop
theorize	suggest, argue
there can be little doubt that	probably
there is . . . , there are . . .	miss out?
treatment modality	treatment
ultimate	final
upon	on
usage (except: language usage)	use
using, utilizing	by, by means of, with
utilize	use
utilization	use
valid	relevant, sound
very	miss out!
while	though, whereas?
with reference to	about
with regard to	in, to, for
x-ray (if the ray itself is not meant!)	x-ray study, picture, examination

References and Further Reading

REFERENCES

WHO 1 = Hogarth J. (1975). *Glossary of Health Care Terminology*. WHO Regional Office for Europe, Copenhagen.

WHO 2 = *International Classification of Impairment, Disabilities and Handicaps* (1980). World Health Organization, Geneva.

SUGGESTED READING

Calnan J., Barabas A. (1973). *Writing Medical Papers – a Practical Guide*. Heinemann, London.

Council of Biology Editors (1983). *CBE Style Manual. A Guide for Authors, Editors, and Publishers in the Biological Sciences*, 5th edn. Council of Biology Editors, Inc., Bethesda, Maryland.

Dirckx J.H. (1976). *The Language of Medicine, Its Evolution, Structure and Dynamics*. Harper & Row, Hagerstown, Pennsylvania.

Lock S. (1977). *Thorne's Better Medical Writing*, 2nd edn. Pitman Medical, Tunbridge Wells, Kent.

O'Connor M., Woodford F.P. (1975). *Writing Scientific Papers in English*. An ELSE-Ciba Foundation Guide for Authors, Elsevier, Amsterdam.